Diyamah A. Rahman
7/95

Women As Wombs

REPRODUCTIVE TECHNOLOGIES AND THE BATTLE OVER WOMEN'S FREEDOM

Janice G. Raymond

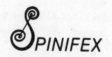

SPINIFEX

Spinifex Press Pty Ltd
504 Queensberry Street
North Melbourne Vic. 3051
Australia

First published in Hardback by HarperSanFrancisco, 1993
This edition published by Spinifex Press, 1994.

FIRST EDITION
Printed in the United States of America

CIP
Raymond, Janice G.
Women as wombs : reproductive technologies and the battle over women's freedom.
Bibliography.
Includes index.
ISBN 1 875559 26 4
1. Human reproductive technology—Moral and ethical aspects.
2. Human reproductive technology—Political aspects.   3. Women—United States—Social conditions.   I. Title.
176

This edition is printed on acid-free paper.

CONTENTS

ACKNOWLEDGMENTS

Over the course of the last seven years of writing this book, many people have generously shared material and experience, sent me various resources, and played a role in the ultimate shaping of this work.

Pat Hynes has been my in-house editor extraordinaire, editing my manuscript in the same way that she edits my life—by being challenging, caring, committed, and brilliantly provocative.

Much of the material that I used was in foreign languages and for their patience in helping me to translate these sources, I thank Rita Arditti, Renate Klein, Michelle Melchionda, Silvia Federici, and my former student Oreli Rodriquez. Additionally, Rita and Silvia sent me many articles that were very helpful. Ahilemah Jonet generously shared all of her sources and writings on international adoption and organ traffiicking.

For other materials and for discussing parts of this book with me, I would also like to thank Brinton Lykes, Lynette Dumble, Margie Hynes, Marysol Asencio, Renée Bridel, and Elise Young. My parents collected numerous newspaper clippings and passed them along at crucial points in the writing. Anne Simon saved me from my inability to grasp the system of legal footnoting and graciously undertook this onerous task, as well as giving me legal advice on various aspects of the writing.

Anita Weigel made my computer behave when I needed to do something beyond basic word processing. And during the last several years, former students such as Barb Nesto, Celeste Friend, and Carol Gomez have tracked down articles and other materials difficult to find.

My friends and colleagues in international FINRRAGE, especially Renate Klein, Robyn Rowland, Jalna Hanmer, Farida Akhter, Ana dos Reis, Rita Arditti, and, most particularly, Gena Corea have supported this work in ways that are both public and personal. Without their courageous writing, organizing, and activism on behalf of women internationally, this book would not be what it is today. I also thank many of the women I worked with during the time that the National Coalition Against Surrogacy was active, especially Pat Mounce, Dianne Rothberg, and Elizabeth Kane.

I thank Kathy Barry for providing me with insight into the area of reproductive trafficking. Other friends have helped in a variety of ways: Andrea Dworkin, Twiss and Pat Butler, and Ronnie Treanor. Mary Daly was especially instrumental in supporting this work.

Finally, I thank my agent, Charlotte Raymond, and my editors at Harper San Francisco, John Loudon and Joanne Moschella, for their help in bringing this manuscript to print.

When I was in graduate school, one of my medical ethics professors asserted that technological reproduction was "at least half a century off." That was 1971; this is 1993. "Half a century off" was also the public's forecast for the advent of reproductive and genetic technologies until scientists publicized their first documented in vitro fertilization (IVF) achievement in 1978. Baby Louise Brown became the world's first technological child, and the planet was put on notice that the technological was made flesh.

In vitro fertilization was the showcase technology in whose glow all the others basked. Billed as a remarkable scientific success, "test-tube babies" legitimated much more. As social psychologist Robyn Rowland has pointed out, in vitro fertilization began the "softening up" process for public acceptance of a long and ever-lengthening line of new reproductive technologies and, eventually, of reproductive contracts:[1] the offshoots of in vitro fertilization such as GIFT (gamete intrafallopian transfer) and ZIFT (zygote intrafallopian transfer); superovulation with fertility drugs; TUDOR (transvaginal ultrasound-directed oocyte recovery); and fetal reduction or selective termination of pregnancy. Other new reproductive technologies and procedures that I critically analyze are sex predetermination; Norplant; embryo transfer; surrogacy;

surrogate gestation; embryo and egg freezing; fetal tissue transplants; and postmortem cesarian sections. A host of other reproductive technologies are now in use, not to mention the wider gamut of genetic technologies being developed for human reproductive purposes, such as genetic screening.

Many of these technologies and contracts will be discussed in this book. In future chapters, I describe what they are, how they work, and what their professed value is. *Professed* is an important word, since part of this book's purpose is to examine the medical and media professions of faith in technological reproduction. Like religious fundamentalism, medical fundamentalism sets up a determining set of beliefs in the efficacy of its own experiments. This book is a challenge to a medicalized *reproductive fundamentalism* that reduces infertility to a disease and promotes the new reproductive technologies and contracts as a cure.

Primarily, this book is a gender-specific analysis of technological and contractual reproduction; that is, it is principally about the consequences of reproductive technologies and contracts for women. Because all these technologies, drugs, and procedures violate the integrity of a woman's body in ways that are dangerous, destructive, debilitating, and demeaning, they are a form of medical violence against women. Some of these, such as reproductive contracts (surrogacy) create a traffic in women's bodies.

Of course, women do not necessarily agree that this is so. Some women have had successful results with these technologies; others believe that these technologies and contracts give women reproductive freedom and choice and enable infertile women to have children. This book disputes these dominant assumptions and addresses, specifically, the feminist controversy over these technologies and contracts. In challenging these procedures as reproductive choice, this book calls into question the going version of procreative liberty and contests that these technologies liberate women.

The international dimension of new reproductive procedures is a consistent theme throughout this work. Much of the current discussion of new reproductive techniques ignores international connections. The debate over surrogacy in the United States is often reduced to issues about contracts, payment, and reproductive rights, as if the consequences of surrogacy are limited to the national domestic sphere.

When surrogacy is validated in the northern hemisphere, however, the baby markets in the developing southern hemisphere, already fueled by northern demand for adoptable children, expand. When medical researchers develop a so-called need for fetal tissue in the West, the trafficking in women and fetuses increases in the East. At the same time that infertility is proclaimed to be epidemic in the industrialized countries, sterilization is rampant in developing countries.

This book is also about language. I highlight the political conse-quences of calling real mothers "surrogate" or substitute mothers, and calling ejaculatory sperm sources "fathers." I discuss a medical dis-course that identifies women as "alternative reproductive vehicles," "maternal environments," and "human incubators." Technological and contractual reproduction degenderizes language and procreation as if women were not involved at all.

Finally, in this book I articulate the connections between sexuality and reproduction in an attempt to bring together sexual and reproduc-tive politics. We cannot continue, for example, to discuss abortion without discussing how and why women become pregnant. And we cannot continue to separate reproductive abuse from the sexual abuse of women. Surrogate contracts and technological reproduction depend upon access to women's bodies, an access that is as sexual as it is re-productive. Those who are concerned about new reproductive pro-cedures cannot afford to reduce them, as do the technoscientists, to a technological problem.

A Question of Choice and Reproductive Rights?

New reproductive arrangements are presented as a woman's private choice. But they are publicly sanctioned violence against women. The absoluteness of this privatized perspective, especially as emphasized by the medical profession and the media, who present women as having unconditioned free will, functions as a smoke screen for medical ex-perimentation and, ultimately, for the violation of women's bodies. Choice so dominates the discourse that it is almost impossible to recog-nize the injury that is done to women.

Choice resonates as a quintessential U.S. value, set in the context of a social history that has gradually allowed all sorts of oppressive so-called options, such as prostitution, pornography, and breast implants, to be defended in the name of women's right to choose. The language of choice is compelling because it highlights a freedom that many women seldom have and a cafeteria of options disguised as self-determination. Viewing reproductive technologies and contracts mainly as a woman's choice results from a particular Western ideology that emphasizes individual freedom and value neutrality. At the same time, this ideology prevents us from examining technological and contractual reproduction as an institution and leads us to neglect the conditions that create industrialized breeding and the role that it plays in society. Choice so dominates the discussion that when critics of technological reproduction denounce the ways in which women are abused by these procedures, we are accused of making women into victims and, supposedly, of denying that women are capable of choice. To expose the victimization of women is to be blamed for creating women as victims.

Whose interests are served by representing technological reproduction as a woman's private choice while rendering invisible the force of institutionalized male-dominant interests? Furthermore, is choice the real issue, or is the issue *what* those choices are and in what context selective women's choices (surrogacy or IVF) are fostered? At the very least, choice implies awareness of possible consequences—what women lack in the reproductive technological and contractual context. At the very most, choice implies that women's health, autonomy, integrity, and basic social justice are served.

Various reproductive rights groups have included within their list of demands access to technological reproduction and surrogacy. Technological reproduction is sometimes defended as part of the pro-choice platform. Borrowing from the abortion defense, reproductive liberals contend that feminists must support these technologies and contracts as part of a woman's right to choose. The right to abortion is combined with the right to reproductive technologies and contracts as a total package that many women feel compelled to accept.

In the supposed interests of women, reproductive liberals have tried to silence critics of technological and contractual reproduction with the accusation that if we speak out against these procedures, we endanger women's reproductive freedom and give arguments to the anti-abortionists. Every criticism of these procedures is linked with the foes of abortion and subjected to the charges of stifling technology, freedom of research, and repressing women's choice. There is a vast difference, however, between women's right to choose safe, legal abortions and women's right to choose unsafe, experimental, and demeaning technologies and contracts. One allows genuine control over the course of a life; the other promotes abdication of control over the self, the body, and reproduction in general. Furthermore, our response to the right wing cannot simply be, "babies made to order." The concept of choice, if it is to have any feminist value, must not be advanced as an absolute right, else it risks reduction to a mere market consumerism.

The subverting of choice by the medical and corporate professionals to promote technological and contractual reproduction has been a largely unexamined area. The rhetoric of choice, however, belies its reality for women. Often what gets promoted as choice, such as the right to choose surrogate contracts, are outright constraints on women's capacity to choose. We cannot continue to pay lip service to reproductive choice while totally ignoring the control that these reproductive arrangements exercise over women.

In this book I contend that those who *support* and *promote* technological and contractual reproduction are *undermining* women's reproductive rights, especially women's right to abortion. The extent to which the rights of women are diminished when the fetus is part of the woman's body—for example, in conservative anti-abortion policy and legislation—should make us seriously question the extent to which they will be further diminished as the fetus is increasingly removed from the female body. Whether in the womb or outside, attention is riveted on the fetus as individual entity—patient, person, or experimentee. IVF; embryo experimentation, transfer, and freezing; and fetal tissue research sever the embryo/fetus from the woman. Reproductive technologies and contracts augment the rights of fetuses and would-be fathers while challenging the one right that women have historically retained some vestige of—mother-right.

We witness this assault on women's rights in surrogate custody disputes and in frozen embryo contests where the rights of "ejaculatory fathers" (see chapter 2) are presented as men's rights to gender equality (or, as the fathers' rights movement phrases it, "Equal rights are not for women only"). These techniques render women as spectators of rather than participants in the whole reproductive process. More and more, they reduce women to the status of vehicle for the fetus; biologically, they literally sunder the fetus from the pregnant woman. Politically and legally, technological reproduction tends to position the fetus as isolated and independent from the mother but not from the sperm source, the doctor, or the state.

The right to choose is fast becoming the right to consume (see chapter 3). Reducing choice to consumption is nothing new. Corporate and professional interests, for many years, have used the rhetoric of choice to sell themselves and their products. What is new is the way in which liberalism and feminism have taken up the language of the corporate world and become consumer movements for new technologies and drugs—in the case of technological reproduction, for more and more dangerous and dubious technologies and drugs. The language of choice makes reproductive consumerism ethical.

This book is a challenge to reproductive liberalism, including its feminist variety. It is positioned against the liberal consumer movement that supports new reproductive technologies and contracts. It is not a balanced approach to both sides of the issue, nor does it provide the supporters of these technologies with equal time. Their position is dominant, well known, and widely publicized (see chapter 3). Radical feminist work on the new reproductive technologies has effectively been censored in both the mainstream media and the mainstream feminist press. This book gives voice to these censored protests.

Challenging Reproductive Fundamentalism

Many people are willing to question a fundamentalism that is overtly religious, yet when these same practices appear in the guise of a secular science, they are not recognized as fundamentalism. Like other fundamentalisms, reproductive fundamentalism has a totalizing capacity. Psychiatrist Robert Jay Lifton has defined totalistic ideology as an exclusive claim to truth by full-blown manipulations of the environment. In analyzing "thought reform" in China, Lifton points to its ability to rehabilitate the individual by controlling specific but unlimited aspects of the person's environment. In *The Nazi Doctors*, Lifton applies this totalizing of the environment to what he calls "medical fundamentalism."

I have used many of these totalizing features[2] as a framework within which to view technological reproduction:

Milieu Control—Scientists and technologists shape public perception of the technologies through what social critics Edward Herman and Noam Chomsky call "manufacturing consent." Favorable press coverage of the technologies is created through a large public relations effort set up by hospitals and research facilities that are adept at marketing these technologies to the public through the media. Images of "miracle" technologies, drugs as "magic bullets," and society on the "frontier" of a "reproductive revolution" pervade the media presentation. Metaphors of progress dominate the coverage, and critical commentary is either ignored or confined to a capsulized space. Critics, who emphasize the political dimensions of medical research and technologies, tend to provide more in-depth analysis and are thus less likely to be quoted. Such critical commentary is not amenable to shrinkage—to the self-promoting sound bites of the scientific public relations enterprise that are so appealing to the media.

Mystical Manipulation—Clinicians represent themselves, and are represented, in the media as white-coated knights, altruistically seeking to help the infertile. "Help for the infertile" has been the dominant meaning given to these technologies. But infertility is a script—what the dictionary defines as a "dialogue spoken in a designated setting"—that was written *after* the technoscientists produced the technological scenario.

The script of infertility—the dialogue of benevolent doctors and desperate couples—came after the fact of technological reproduction, not before it. As Erwin Chargaff, a noted molecular biologist, has stated, "The demand [for the technologies] was less overwhelming than the desire on the part of the scientists to test their newly developed techniques. The experimental babies produced were more of a by-product."[3] Chargaff's view is supported by reports that over 200,000 embryos have been stockpiled in European IVF centers that have been specifically created for research.[4]

Sacred Science—Technological reproduction is mystified as the greatest hope for the infertile. Reproductive experts highlight successes and omit the numbers of failed attempts. The most blatant example of this misrepresentation is the reported IVF success rates in which success is often measured by the number of chemical pregnancies (hormone levels that may indicate pregnancy but are frequently false positives) and pregnancies per laparoscopy, many of which do not issue in live births.[5] As surprising as this revelation has been to people, a large number of IVF clinics still do not measure success by numbers of live births. Many people do not know that the IVF success rate is between 0 percent and 15 percent, depending on the clinic. IVF success has been highest in Australia, yet a 1988 Australian government study found that "there is no evidence that IVF has had a higher success rate than other treatments for infertility, or even that it has a higher success rate than the absence of all treatment."[6]

Loading of the Language—Medical and media claims that technological reproduction is a "cure for infertility" become a cliché that suppresses critical questioning. Unpacking this claim requires acknowledging that technological reproduction and surrogate contracts do not cure infertility but only provide some (mostly white, middle-class, married, heterosexual) couples with children and then, only a very small percentage of the time. Terms such as *surrogate mother* and *biological father* spawn new definitions of motherhood and fatherhood and stymy critical thinking about what the words mean. In the 1987 Baby M surrogacy case, the constant repetition of *surrogate mother* and *biological father*, like a mantra, helped confirm that Mary Beth Whitehead was a mere substitute rather than a real mother, while Bill Stern became the real parent rather than a sperm source. Stern's victory—being awarded custody of the child—was partly one of language. At other times, Stern was represented as simply the "father," and Whitehead as the "surrogate mother." She became the modified parent diminished by a qualifying adjective; his parenthood was straightforward—simply "father." The term *surrogate* reduces all women who sign surrogate contracts to incidental, nonparental status.

The new reproductive language is loaded in other ways. Are the deaths of women in IVF programs "unfortunate incidents" or "medical disasters"? Does it make a difference if Clomid, a hormone used to superovulate women on IVF programs to produce multiple eggs,[7] is called a "potential risk" rather than a "debilitating drug"? Is the past history of reproductive drug and technology failures—as represented by thalidomide, diethylstilbestrol (DES), and estrogen replacement therapy, for example—"aberrant" or "typical"? Some words imply judgments; others convey value neutrality. Some trivialize an event; others highlight its significance. Choice of adjectives can marginalize some opinions while giving authority to others. Some words endow a technology with public stature; others diminish its status.

Doctrine over Person—Women's experiences of self, of reproduction, and of pregnancy are subsumed or negated by the system of technological reproduction. Women are not present in the medical language, which speaks only of "maternal environments" and "alternative reproductive vehicles." In the popular discourse about surrogacy, women who enter into surrogate arrangements have called themselves "baby-sitters" for "other people's children." Worse still, women are not present to themselves. One woman, passed along the in vitro fertilization production line, describes herself in the third person:

> Here she is . . . debased and degraded, embarrassed and humbled, shamed and subdued. Their guinea-pig, their hatching-hen, hormone cow, their willing victim. And why? Because, fifteen years ago, when all she willed was sex and not babies, the doctor put an IUD in her almost virgin womb. . . .[8]

Closely connected with the absence of self is *the dispensing of existence* experienced by women in technological reproduction. Time, relationships, jobs are dispensed with. Women undergoing these procedures report a sense of nonbeing:

> A broken vessel. A barren land. An empty shell. A nothingness, a nullity, a non-being.[9]

This dispensing of existence is more than psychological and existential. Women on in vitro fertilization programs have literally died, and at least one woman lost her life while bearing a surrogate pregnancy from complications directly resulting from callous negligence of her heart condition by the broker—who was a real estate agent—and the doctor to whom she was sent.[10]

As in other fundamentalisms, certain beliefs and principles are basic to the system of technological reproduction. The first principle is that *infertility is a disease for which reproductive technology is the remedy*. If doctors are curing a disease, then much becomes acceptable.

As cultural critic Susan Sontag has stated, "The concept of disease is never innocent."[11] Paraphrasing Sontag, to describe a phenomenon as a disease is an "incitement" to the development of a technology (see chapter 1). Technology, whether constructive or destructive, is construed as therapy. It is time, however, to reverse this popular wisdom and ask whether reproductive technology is itself the disease, the disease of chronic medicalization of women's bodies, often engendering a string of problems that are worse than anything caused by the original symptom of infertility.

A second principle of technological reproduction is that *reproduction is mainly a technical problem*. Technology comes to dominate the field of attention, not only in the medical literature, but in the popular articles devoted to disseminating the good news of reproductive salvation. Explanations of the wizardry of new procedures that promise a coming of fertility and doctor-as-hero stories inundate us with facts and figures. Medical generals are presented to the public in ways comparable to the U.S. media reporting of the war against Iraq. The medical literature renders hyperstimulation of the ovaries and cysts, a frequent by-product of superovulation used in IVF, into a mere technological imperfection of the procedure—"collateral damage" as it is called in war, signifying any destruction outside the intended parameters of the target: "We never meant to burst your ovaries." Likewise, women are not told that most of these reproductive technologies are still in the experimental stage.

As a technological problem, *reproduction requires a professional elite* to solve it. Yet there is no official board certification for a fertility specialist. Any doctor may hang out such a shingle, and by all reports, they are hanging them out at a fast clip. Between 1974 and 1988, membership in the American Fertility Society jumped from 3,600 to 10,300.[12] The most ordinary of scientists, most notably animal specialists, become world-renowned human reproductive virtuosos.

Jacques Testart, technodaddy of France's first IVF baby, Amandine; director of research at the National Institute of Health and Medical Research in Paris; and now avatar of medical ethics for renouncing his own human IVF research, began his career as an animal biologist. He started as an expert in the superfecundation of cattle and the transfer of genetically selected embryos into surrogate mother cows. After leaving the farm, he came to the big city of Paris and began applying his animal research to women.

Likewise, Alan Trounson of Australian IVF repute started his work as a sheep embryologist. He then applied this knowledge to human IVF treatment. In a remarkable turnaround, Trounson took what he had learned on women with the Monash IVF team and now uses a similar technology to breed goats. According to news reports, Trounson, who is now director of International Breeding and Technology located in Rye, close to the Monash Medical Centre at Clayton, is implanting ordinary feral goats with the embryos of purebred Angora goats, using the former as surrogate gestators.[13]

At surrogacy trials and in other court cases such as the Tennessee embryo-freezing dispute, a professional elite, who often has a history of collaboration with the surrogate brokers and lawyers, is also called upon to testify. Increasingly, reproductive decisions become adjudicated by these professional experts. In the Baby M case, experts who were mainly psychologists supposedly measured Mary Beth Whitehead's fitness for motherhood. Using a positivistic methodology, they pronounced on the appropriateness of Whitehead giving her child panda bears versus pots and pans. Because Whitehead had presented her baby with the so-called wrong toys, she was judged an unfit mother. These reputedly learned experts lent the pro-Stern forces a measured superiority. Furthermore, the transformation of surrogacy from a dubious idea to accepted public policy has been achieved primarily through expert testimony from specialists and practitioners appearing before legislative committees.

This professional elite, however, is not a unified group. Researchers and clinicians, as well as surrogate brokers, question each other's credentials by pointing out the competition's lack of quality control. Bill Handel, a surrogate broker in California, complains that Noel Keane's screening procedures are sloppy, that his operation is lowbrow, and that Mary Beth Whitehead never would have passed muster in Handel's center. "Keane will take anybody who walks through the door,"[14] Handel has said, even those women who have been screened out by Keane's own employed psychologists.[15] In a more low-key manner, IVF experts imply that misreporting of IVF success rates comes from competition for clients and publicity, but that their own clinics are top-notch.[16]

Another fundamental principle operating in the defense of technological reproduction is that *persons have a biological need to reproduce.* Terms like *genetic continuity, biological fulfillment, reproductive imperative,* and *maternal instinct* mystify motherhood and fatherhood, detracting from our ability to recognize them as personal and social relationships. When male claims to children are asserted, as in surrogacy disputes, we hear about men's right to genetic "fulfillment."[17] When new technological procedures are launched for public acceptance, we hear about "women's natural need" to reproduce. Patrick Steptoe, lab parent of the world's first IVF baby, asserted, "It is a fact that there is a biological drive to reproduce. Women who deny this drive, or in whom it is frustrated, show disturbances in other ways."[18]

What defenders of new reproductive techniques regard as natural, feminists challenge as political. As feminists have attacked the false essentialism that the male sexual urge is uncontrollable and therefore men need prostitutes to satisfy their sexual needs, so too feminists oppose the idea that reproduction is a biological imperative. Feminists challenge men's need for so-called surrogates in order to fulfill their supposed genetic destiny of fathering children. Technological reproduction has also been grounded in women's need for children, thus providing the excuse for many invasive and mutilating procedures. It is rationalized that women who submit to such techniques are fulfilling their basic mothering instinct. In both examples, anything a man or woman does to procreate is a natural urge, an instinctual force, that must have an outlet. The difference is that men do not usually consent to their own exploitation but to the exploitation of a woman, whereas a woman undergoing invasive reproductive medicine must submit to a violation of her own bodily integrity, even if she consents to the procedure.

Since the nineteenth century especially, the so-called laws of nature have come to be understood more and more in scientific terms. Scientists analyze, dissect, and categorize what were formerly natural or divine dictums such as racial and gender differences. Procreation is perceived as a law of nature that, in the context of new reproductive technologies, acquires an expanded scientific mandate. Scientific legitimacy makes it more difficult to challenge the medical model of procreation as a natural law demanding fulfillment.

At this historical point when feminists have de-essentialized motherhood—politicizing the natural definition of women as mothers and distinguishing between motherhood as experience and motherhood as institution—along come the reproductive medical fundamentalists to put mothering back into the sphere of women's natural destiny. The new reproductive technologies represent an appropriation by male scientific experts of the female body, depoliticizing reproduction and motherhood by recasting these roles as fundamental instincts that must be satisfied.

An Issue of Violence Against Women

Many feminists contend that the new reproductive technologies are a form of medical violence against women. Others say this contention is "going too far," yet they do not regard what women are required to submit to as "going too far." I maintain in this book that much of technological reproduction is brutality with a therapeutic face.

As the nineteenth- and early twentieth-century sexologists promoted a theory of female masochism that collapsed sexual pain with sexual pleasure for women, the reproductive technologists operate on a similar principle that women will accept any pain to create a child. The religious version of this principle was articulated by Martin Luther when he said that the more pain a woman suffers in childbirth, the more she will love the child. Its secular version is another fundamental of technological reproduction: women are willing to suffer any pain, any invasive procedure, any medical violence to become pregnant.

With sex, many women have been forced or wooed into compliance. "*You will* do this," or "*Will you* do this for me?" "Will you do this for me?" says the infertile husband whose often fertile wife becomes the IVF patient—one of the only situations in medicine where the person treated is not the person with the problem. Women's acceptance of these invasive and damaging procedures to conceive a child, whether from their own desire, their husband's, or both, has blunted the medical violence intrinsic to the procedures.

If a person is violated medically in an experiment, in a prison, or for political reasons, people respond with outrage. But if a woman is violated medically, in the interests of helping her to reproduce, it is justified as therapeutic; people dismiss it as a benevolent treatment for infertility—her own or her partner's. For the reproductive experts, infertility therapy covers a multitude of medical violations. Women are told if they want babies, put up with the pain, the humiliation, the stress, and maybe they'll get one. They are not told, but it is inherent in IVF treatment, that they must also put up with, among other things, hyperstimulation of the ovaries, possible cysts, and the procedure of having to eliminate multiple fetuses in utero after superovulation. They are certainly not told about the women who have died on IVF programs. Doctors minimize and even censor the brutality of the technologies, the medical casualties, and of course the body count.

H. Patricia Hynes, an environmental engineer, has compared the existence of embryo protection legislation in certain countries to the nonexistence of legislation protecting the women whose bodies are used in these very same procedures.

> In many countries experimentation on embryos is limited to the first 14 days of life. In those same countries experimentation on women with risk-laden drugs and medical procedures is not limited or forestalled. . . . Embryos, it seems, are better protected than women from invasive and potentially dangerous technologies.[19]

Technological reproduction creates an environment of medical experimentation in which virtually anything can be tried on women's bodies. The claims that the technology is being perfected all the time camouflages the medicalized mutilation inherent in the procedures. In the medical literature, there is also a "violence of abstraction," where what is done to women is encased in "numbers of pregnancies per laparoscopy" or "selective therapeutic termination of pregnancy." But women are not abstract, and neither are the mutilations inflicted on women's bodies.

Making International Connections

Most discussion of contractual and technological reproduction in the West is confined to national boundaries. The way in which these technologies have been framed as a consumer choice is but one example. Additionally, much of the scientific commentary focuses on the techniques, their relative merits, the developing science or medicine that promises more and more, and the potential of the technology to cure an ever-expanding repertoire of diseases. The legal literature is fixated on patents, contracts, competing interests of the parties involved, access, and issues of rights. The ethical literature seems to dwell on blaming women for the current moral dilemmas posed by the new technologies.

Unnoticed in most discussions of technological reproduction and reproductive contracts is the creation of a new form of *reproductive trafficking*—the international medical research networks; the international markets for women used in surrogacy, fetal tissue, and eggs; the global stockpiling of frozen embryos; the technology transfers; and the increasing exchange of human material from one woman to another. The reproductive use and abuse of women is being played out on an international medical stage where women's bodies, children, and fetuses are being trafficked across national borders.

The trafficking in women and children for sex has been and still is a restricted topic of discussion. Likewise, the trafficking in women for reproduction and the children who are produced is even more hidden. I refer here to women used in developing countries to produce babies for individual foreigners or for foreign adoptions, usually in the West; and women kept on literal "baby farms" or who hire out privately, delivering the baby to a middleman who then completes the transaction with an individual or agency in a developed country. There are many variations on this trafficking, which will be discussed in a later chapter. Trafficking also includes fetal tissue imported from abroad or obtained from abortion clinics in the West, whether harvested without women's consent from elective abortions or from direct payment to women who conceive in order to abort because they need the money.

Finally, there is the murky world of children or children's organs exported for transplants in the industrialized countries. The trade in organs taken from children in developing countries is very much related to reproductive trafficking because it follows the sexual and reproductive trafficking routes; it is intimately allied with the commerce in children for adoption; it has a medical foundation; and it is increasingly viewed in international and United Nations circles as a development in contemporary forms of trafficking. For example, the 1991 *Report of the Working Group on Contemporary Forms of Slavery,* part of a UN sub-commission on Prevention of Discrimination and Protection of Minorities, at its sixteenth session, for the first time reviewed allegations of child organ trafficking in connection with the international sexual trafficking in women and children and the worldwide adoption traffic.[20]

Organ trafficking has also been the most difficult form of traffic in persons and persons' body parts to prove, stonewalled by silence and the reluctance of governments and individuals to investigate. Additionally, suppression of evidence about the complete network of reproductive trafficking has been justified by the so-called medical need for organ transplants, fetal tissue research, legal surrogacy, and the demand for adoptable babies in the West (see chapter 5).

Reproductive contracts and techniques, such as surrogate arrangements, have also created a *national traffic* in women exploited for their reproductive faculties and functions. Literally, this is a system in which women are movable property, objects of exchange, brokered by go-betweens mainly serving the buyer. Surrogate contracts are not simply individual arrangements between women and supposedly desperate couples. They are reproductive purchase orders where women are *procured* as instruments in a system of breeding. The language and reality of surrogacy as *reproductive trafficking* cuts through its accepted image as a simple contractual agreement between giving women and despondent couples. In the Third World, they call this procurement baby farming; in the First World, they call it surrogacy.

The distinction between surrogacy and baby farming is collapsed by surrogate brokers who quite candidly admit that they will seek new and more inexpensive markets for breeders and babies in developing countries, where they will procure women for what are now referred to as "intrauterine adoptions." A surrogate broker in the United States has acknowledged that he will increasingly turn to Third World countries for his stable of women breeders since, he says, the going rate will be cheaper and the labor supply more unquestioning.[21] Also, the specter of international reproductive exploitation has become so serious that the vulnerability of women in developing countries at risk for "womb renting" was raised at the 1992 Committee on the Elimination of Discrimination Against Women (CEDAW) hearings at the United Nations.[22]

Intercountry adoption is closely allied with surrogacy. Often referred to as "The Baby Trade," international adoption is an already established reproductive trafficking that has existed for years. In proposing an alternative to technological reproduction, we cannot state so glibly that persons should adopt so-called unwanted Third World babies. Many of these children are very much wanted but have been *taken* from women, families, and cultures.

The various ways in which children are procured for adoption forms a separate chapter in this book (see chapter 5). But one thing is clear: Western demand for adoptable children from abroad exceeds legal supply. In Guatemala, the exporting of children has become the primary cash crop of the country, much of it the result of U.S. involvement in Central America. The adoption traffic moves from the less developed to the more developed countries, "from poor women toward rich men, in all directions."[23] Many children adopted—even under legal conditions in the West and North—are procured, kidnapped, or stolen from women (see chapter 5). The falsification of the child's birth certificate is said to be the easiest part of the adoption process. Other children who end up in the adoption trade are the result of pregnancies caused by rape during war.

The reproductive use and abuse of women is also played out on the international stage of population policy and programs. In contrast to the technologies and drugs promoting fertility, which are now common in the so-called First World, Third World women receive drugs and technologies designed to promote infertility. Repeated sterilization and the exporting of dangerous contraceptives are the consequences of technological reproduction for women in Third World countries. If infertility is genuinely the concern of medical science, why is medical science not doing something to stop the greatest cause of infertility in the world—mass sterilization of women in developing countries? The question is rhetorical. Medical science and technology are promoting infertility in the Third World while denouncing it in the First World.

Third World countries have been a past and present dumping ground for chemicals and drugs banned in the West—DDT and DES, for example. Now these countries are testing sites for a new and unproven rash of hormonal and chemical contraceptives such as Norplant, the surgical implant that remains embedded under a woman's skin for about five years. When Norplant was first tested in Brazil and Bangladesh, women experienced harmful complications. Women's groups and health organizations in both countries campaigned against the trials (see chapter 1).

The rationale that female fertility is out of control in the Third World has also generated another and more drastic supposed solution—sex predetermination. When population control proves too sluggish, exterminate the root of the problem—women. Women have long been viewed as population polluters in the Third World, and for the last twenty years some scientists have proposed that they reduce the number of women born—selective termination of female fetuses or, as the reality has been in many parts of India, *massive termination of female fetuses.* Between the years 1978 and 1983, 78,000 female fetuses are estimated to have been aborted following clinical amniocentesis in India.[24] A study of 8,000 cases of abortion in Bombay also revealed that 7,997 of the fetuses were female.[25]

In India, the widespread use of amniocentesis for sex predetermination has been used for over a decade. Doctors were quick to realize its potential in detecting the sex of the fetus, and sex predetermination clinics were thus set up and widely advertised in many Indian cities, towns, and suburbs. The inexpensiveness of the test meant that it became available to all classes, and government support initially assured it would not be banned. Vibuti Patel, political activist and economist, contrasts this support for amniocentesis for purposes of sex predetermination with the failure of the government to support amniocentesis for pregnant women during the Bhopal chemical disaster and its aftermath, "in spite of repeated requests by women's groups and in spite of many reported cases of the birth of deformed babies as a result of the gas carnage."[26]

In this book I underscore the international connections of reproductive technologies not only to document and analyze the global dimensions of the expanding reproductive supermarket, but also to chronicle the most powerful and successful feminist responses and challenges to these technologies. The political activism of Indian women has been instrumental in bringing about new legislation that prohibits using amniocentesis for sex predetermination in parts of India (chapter 1). In the otherwise bleak picture of the state of technological reproduction, the Indian women's campaign and their limited success stands as an example to feminists in the West. Theirs has been a feminist victory for all women who recognize the subversion of women's choice for opportunistic medical gains, and for all women who know the difference between choice and its constraints.

The Sexualization of Reproduction

The debates about abortion, contraception, reproductive rights, and reproductive technologies often take place without considering how and why women become pregnant. Reproduction is sexual, whether in the bedroom or the laboratory. Feminists cannot advocate for reproductive freedom without advocating that women control their sexuality. Critics of abortion restrictions, for example, cannot ignore the reason many women need abortions to begin with: because they cannot say no, because they have sex forced on them, because they are raped, because they are prostituted, because they are girls held hostage and made pregnant in families where fathers, brothers, or male relatives use them sexually, because they are teenagers who have sex but do not know why, and because of all the other conditions set in a context of female sexual subordination in which many girls and women "get knocked up." The term itself makes the point.

Reproduction is the consequence of men's sexual access to women. Reproductive abuse of women's bodies is accepted as normal, because sexual abuse has paved the way. Reproductive technologies are the next step enhancing male access to women and the increasing abuse of women's bodies under the guise of scientific advancement. Women are required to spread their legs too frequently for medical probing and penetration.

The industrialization of reproduction moves the issue of access to women's bodies even further beyond what is commonly called the private sphere. Technological reproduction is not only part of the politics of reproduction, but of sexual politics too, for it is primarily about access to women and abuse of women's bodies—for medical research and experimentation, for financial gain, for clinical experience and adventure, for the manipulation of life.

Feminist theory has engendered a debate about the centrality of sexual versus reproductive politics in women's lives. For example, Mary

O'Brien in *The Politics of Reproduction* has asserted that feminist theory should begin "within the process of human reproduction. Of that process, sexuality is but a part."[27] In this book I refuse to confine sexuality to a mere part of reproduction. I assert instead that sexual politics is the basis for any substantive feminist reproductive politics because it raises the crucial issues of access to and abuse of women's bodies. Nor is women's control of sexuality merely the freedom from state regulation and repressive ideology. It is the freedom from male definition, abuse, and access, institutionalized in what G. J. Barker-Benfield has called the "spermatic economy."[28]

In the spermatic economy of sex and breeding, woman exists for sex. She also exists to become pregnant and reproduce, when and if men want children. There is but a short distance from fucking to breeding in the patriarchal picture. In the spermatic economy of sex and breeding, men spend themselves and their vital, life-giving fluid in sex and are entitled to get it back. Whether as sexual object or reproductive instrument, women are there to give to men. When women cannot serve as natural reproductive instruments, or when men cannot perform their natural fertilizing role, the great technological fuck takes over.

The connection between sexual and reproductive politics is material; that is, it is no mere metaphor. Men have overtly sexualized many reproductive technologies. In 1980, Diana Scully published her book, *Men Who Control Women's Health: The Education of Obstetricians and Gynecologists.* Among the questions she asked, while interviewing practicing physicians and medical students preparing to enter these fields, was what it is like to treat infertility.

> I think it's a big kick to get her pregnant. . . . The girls . . . who get pregnant think that we are great. . . . The husband ends up, at least in the wife's eyes, as playing a very insignificant role. Almost as if the doctor was in bed with her on that fateful night rather than the husband.[29]

Jacques Testart of French IVF fame compares his technological success to an intellectual orgasm. In *L'oeuf transparent* (The Transparent Egg), an account of his own experience working on the French IVF team, Testart describes the process as an intrusion into sexual privacy, a "violation of love and intimacy." The laboratory exposes the woman's womb to the light of day. The dark night of sex becomes the wide-awake day of breaking sexual taboos. As one reviewer noted, the book, written in a provocative style, also describes the easygoing and eroticized manner in which the medical residents go about their fertility business.[30]

Testart further writes of his "incestuous" feelings for his IVF child, Amandine.

> I invested myself in a role that was not . . . paternal. I felt I was the lover, not the father. . . . I would like to discover her once she's become a person. . . . That's why I see myself more as a lover and not as a father.[31]

His assumption of fatherhood is questionable enough; more outrageous is his candid admission of sexual fantasy with an egg/fetus/baby he clearly imagines as his lover. Testart also makes clear that the technologies are about penetration.

In 1869, Josephine Butler condemned enforced medical examination of prostitutes mandated by the Contagious Diseases Acts just enacted in England. She called the exam "instrumental rape" by the "steel penis." Those words apply today to the constant poking and prying—the scientific penetration of women's bodies—especially in the in vitro fertilization context. Take, for example, the way in which eggs are collected from a woman's ovaries for use in IVF procedures. Describing the vaginal harvesting of eggs from a woman's follicles in full view of a class of medical students, a female student-observer of the IVF procedure wrote,

> At each follicle puncture he [the doctor] retracted the needle and then drove it in hard—a movement very similar to the act of penetration. . . . After the fifth follicle had been sucked out, the woman asked him to stop, because she was in great pain. But Dr. M. would have none of that . . . and so the sixth and seventh follicles were punctured against her will. . . . Again each puncture unmistakably resembled a penetration.[32]

Surrogacy is another reproductive procedure that has been overtly sexualized. Women who sign surrogate contracts speak about being wined, dined, and dated by the sperm source. Sexual seductiveness has been a part of the ritual initiated by sperm sources who conduct "romantic" relationships with "their surrogates" during the pregnancy. Some wives of men who hire women as breeders perceive the arrangement not only as men contracting for a surrogate mother but for a surrogate wife. At 1988 Wisconsin state hearings on proposed surrogacy legislation, one woman married to a man who hired a woman was asked how she, as his wife, had experienced the arrangement. Since she had testified several minutes before about the great merits of surrogacy, many were shocked when she sobbed, "It's so humiliating to have my husband ask a strange woman to bear his child."[33]

More and more, the old sexual roles within which women have been confined converge with the new reproductive roles women are offered. Men buying women for sex in prostitution bears striking resemblance to men buying women's reproductive services in surrogacy. Surrogate brokers become reproductive pimps. The men who hire women as surrogates will pay extra for their own specific reproductive proclivities. Some want women inseminated only with sperm bearing the y chromosome; some demand the women undergo amniocentesis for quality control of the product; some want several tricks for the price of one, so they submit the women to superovulation as a hedge that at least one of the resulting multiple eggs will be fertilized.

Surrogate insemination is also seen as a sexual act. In the spermatic economy, pregnancy marks a woman as a man's sexual possession. She is marked by his access to her. In surrogacy, the husbands of contracting women often must give permission for "their" women to be marked by other men. They must also abdicate their rights to the fruit of their wives' wombs. That insemination is indeed regarded as a sexual act is described by exsurrogate Elizabeth Kane in recounting her husband's experience of her surrogate insemination.

> Kent had sunk into the massive leather chair, pretending he didn't know it was time for the insemination. He took a long, slow drink from the glass of wine, avoiding my eyes and fooling no one. . . . With a straight back I walked through the door, away from my husband, to conceive another man's child.[34]

He would be fine, he said, as long as he didn't have to meet the sperm source.

Increasingly, there is a pornography of pregnancy in which women's pregnant bodies, prone bodies, bodies on all fours with ass in air ready for embryo implantation, and bodies with legs up and head down are all portrayed on national TV to show the public how IVF works. This is educational pornography—women in the graphic state of technological manhandling for all the world to watch. As sociologist Jalna Hanmer has stated, "At last I have discovered what the term mother-fucker means and who the mother-fuckers are."[35]

Women are not supposed to be outraged and disturbed by these demeaning images; they are all in the service of technological education. But this is education once more over women's bodies—reproductively prone, vulnerable, ever-accessible women's bodies, with the medical instrument serving as phallus. The completely or seminaked pregnant woman's body among hardly virginal white-clothed men is the new educational graphic for technological reproduction. This is one more variation on the pornography of pregnancy opening the vagina, the pregnant uterus, and the woman herself for viewing.

Pornography is essential in surrogate agencies to help men masturbate for sperm. Kathleen King, another woman who ended up as one of surrogate broker Noel Keane's botched deals, describes her initial awareness that she had been violated: "When I went to New York for the insemination, I accidentally went into the men's bathroom and there were pornography books all over the place. . . ."[36] For King, the pornography served as a vivid illustration of how her own body was being objectified and used.

In the international prostitution industry, marriage catalogs display pictures of women for sale as mail order brides or as sexual servants. In the United States, many surrogate agencies offer clients pictures of women willing to serve as surrogates, often along with children they have produced, so that the customer can see the kind of "stock" he is buying. While these photos are not pornography, there is a link between these pictures and the pornography used by men to produce sperm. As sociologist Louise Vandelac has written, "There is an interesting sort of pornographic continuum, which begins with one man choosing a catalogue mother and ejaculating with a little inspiration provided by 'suggestive' photographs of other women, so that another man can inseminate the initial 'photo-woman.'"[37]

The actual insemination of Elizabeth Kane was pictured in *People* magazine. Repelled by the prospect of being photographed during the insemination, Kane was motivated, that is, pressured into it, by Dr.

Richard Levin, the director of Surrogate Parenting Associates in Louis-ville, Kentucky. "A male photographer from *People* magazine was pres-ent during the entire insemination, promising me it would never be published but was for Dr. Levin's personal photo album only. A full page picture of myself with my legs spread, shaking hands with the insemi-nating nurse, graces the pages of *People*, April 14, 1980."[38] The *People* photographer defended the picture taking and the publishing of it on the grounds that "it's the focal point of the whole story."[39] Why photo-graphs of women being inseminated would be the focal point of the story is a mystery unless the men looking at the photographs found it to be so. Certainly, this would not be a woman's focal point.

There is, in fact, a sense of pornography to the whole process of surrogacy and other new reproductive techniques. Women undergoing IVF treatment talk of feeling objectified, denigrated, and humiliated as they become the embodiments of a medical tutorial for resident physi-cians learning the technique. Exposed to medical viewing, feet in the stirrups, and not in control of themselves or the process, they report feeling like bodies on display. "Supine on the gynecological chair with legs raised and apart she [the woman undergoing the IVF procedure] was trembling with shame and fear—a mere object: available to all those around her."[40] Doctors add to the exposure, often by making comments that promote the sexual objectification of the experience for the woman. One woman, on display in the stirrups for visiting doctors from IVF programs around the world, was playfully told by her doctor that she would have an "international fanny." The implication was that she would somehow be thrilled at being seen by these international doctors, when the reality was that they were titillated at seeing her with "a huge spotlight shining on [her] genitals."[41]

Women who have signed surrogate contracts and who have had the courage to fight back legally speak about their humiliation and objecti-fication when they appear in a public forum. The so-called surrogate physically embodies her protest. Exposed to public view, she becomes a centerfold who is marked negatively by what is regarded by many as a kind of prostitute pregnancy. The legal process renders her exposed, like a woman in pornography, graphically depicting her as reproductive whore. This defines her, this objectifies her, and her pain is turned into others' pleasure.

Infertility is the new frigidity in which women's bodies are viewed as unable (unwilling) to reproduce. As defined by the early twentieth-century sexologists, frigidity was woman's failure to respond with enthusiasm to heterosexual intercourse. Many experts believed that the so-called problem of frigidity was intractable in many middle- and upper-class women of the day and required the physician's intervention "whose 'prescription' was essentially an attempt to force the wife to do what the husband had been unable to make her do—to submit."[42] In the same way that frigidity required "educating the vagina" to the husband's phallus, infertility requires "educating the uterus" to the husband's (or donor's) sperm fertilized with her (or a donor's) egg. Technology becomes the new instrumental manipulation that will coax women's reluctant bodies into reproductive performance.

Technological reproduction completes the medicalization of sex begun in the nineteenth century. The sexual objectification and violation of women is made invisible because technological reproduction has turned medicalized pornography into education, made medicalized access to the female body acceptable, and transformed medicalized abuse into standard treatment. Technological reproduction is first and foremost about the appropriation of the female body.

For feminists attending the Seventh World Congress on In Vitro Fertilization and Assisted Procreations held in Paris during June and July 1991, this sexualization of reproduction was played out on a literal stage. As part of the inaugural ceremonies marking the beginning of the World Congress, and in the august conference hall of the Palais de Congrès, worldwide IVF practitioners and human reproductive specialists were treated to a bevy of semiclad female dancers performing the French can-can. To the whistles and cheers of the esteemed IVF practitioners, the dancers moved forward to the edge of the stage, first thrusting their pelvises out and then, after withdrawing to the back of the stage, coming forward again with asses thrust out toward their overwhelmingly appreciative male medical audience.

As women, and as feminist critics of the technologies standing at the back of the huge auditorium watching both the dancers and the doctors, we speculated what this performance represented for men who see women in their offices, clinics, and operating theaters in precisely these postures. For one thing, a blurring takes place between images of the female patients in their offices and clinics and the women on the stage—from reproductive to sexual object. What this represented for us standing at the back of the hall was quite different. Women's bodies, once more, were blatantly displayed and easily accessible to men who were reveling in this staged circus of what one of the Parisian hosts described as "the ultimate female bodies."[43] The Seventh World IVF Congress can-can gave the sexual/reproductive game away, revealing that within this system, the main options for women are as sexual or reproductive beings.

Prior to this show of female bodies, we had been examining the new technologies of the multinational reproductive industry as it plied its wares to the fertility doctors, clinicians, and researchers in attendance. We had just been treated to a display of laparoscopes, vaginoscopes, and laser hysteroscopes, many of which were pictured penetrating and probing a woman's reproductive interior. Moving from this exhibition of female flesh to another one—the can-can performance—was like a scene straight out of the film *Dead Ringers*, in which twin gynecologists sexually swap their patients, put women in the stirrups while engaging in sex, and use their gynecological instruments to produce female pain (pleasure). I hissed to the colleague next to me, "No one will ever be able to tell me these technologies have nothing to do with sexual access to women."

Increasingly, in feminist and biomedical circles, reproductive technologies and contracts are debated not only as if they have nothing to do with sexual access to women but as if they have nothing to do with women at all—as if they are mere ideas or academic exercises. Much of this supposed debate represents a combination of drift and dispassion; the debaters explore doubts, suggest inadequacies, but do not make these doubts and inadequacies palpable. Debaters also perform balancing acts, often suggesting *potential* abuse but more interested in defending the use value of these technologies. Frequently, feminists "debate" about whether these technologies are not *simply* abusive to women but can be used by women as well, as if we all need lessons in the complexity and nuances of violation. In the postmodernist world of social criticism in which essays, books, and conference papers have taken on the role of distanced commentary, it is my hope that this book will be a dose of reality. Feminism is only real if it is continuously involved in women's lives.

This book is the result of years of working internationally as an activist with women from different countries against the development and legalization of many of these technologies. In the course of this work, I have come to know many women whose lives have been ravaged by the techniques: exsurrogates who have had the courage to testify against the contracts in the public forum; women who have gone through IVF programs and have experienced physical harms and false hopes; and women who have been sterilized and subjected to contraceptive abuse.

This book is also the result of an academic life, a good portion of which has been spent documenting in the most rigorous way I know the liabilities of these technologies for women. It is my hope that this book will bring together the work of both documentation and advocacy to demonstrate how and why reproductive fundamentalism and its product, reproductive technologies and contracts, are more peril than progress.

CHAPTER ONE

The Production of Fertility and Infertility: East and West, South and North

Technological reproduction is a case study in the politics of both fertility and infertility. In the industrialized countries of the West and the North, it is *infertility* that is of concern to the reproductive experts who tell us that infertility rates are skyrocketing. Infertility is to the twentieth-century Western medical profession what hysteria was to nineteenth-century doctors. It justifies invasive medical intervention, drugs, and surgery on women "for our own good." By medicalizing infertility in the West and North, reproductive experts bring the condition under medical control.

In the East and in the developing South, it is *fertility* that is of concern to the reproductive experts. Population groups and, most recently, environmental organizations, point to Third World fertility rates that are supposedly out of control. This perception of unrestrained female fertility justifies invasive medical intervention—contraceptives, sterilization, and, most recently, sex predetermination used on women in developing countries. Through programs of population planning, fertility is brought under government and medical auspices.

In both areas of the world, however, the common victim and target of medical manipulation is women. It is women who bear the burden of their own and their male partners' infertility in the so-called First

World, and their own and their male partners' fertility in the so-called Third World. In the industrialized reproductive centers of the West, men often do not undergo fertility testing, never mind fertility treatment. In the East, men do not bear the burden of dangerous contraceptives, nor are they, for the most part, subjected to sterilization. In India, where massive male sterilization was tried in the 1970s, the government vasectomy program was so unpopular that it helped drive Indira Gandhi out of office and was discontinued under her successor.[1] Additionally, female sterilization is a much more complicated procedure fraught with major complications.

The *production* of fertility and infertility, that is, the ways in which both are created and commodified as medical problems, is very much linked with the production of distinctively different technologies developed for use in different parts of the world. The ideology of infertility in the West is based on a double standard. Children who are technologically conceived at high cost in the industrialized world—a staggering cost to women's well-being and a high economic cost—are the potential children whose conception is thwarted in the Third World, through sterilization, harmful contraceptives, and sex predetermination, not to mention the existing children who die of poverty, malnutrition, and other causes. Keeping First-Third World connections in view enables us not to lose sight of the global picture of technological reproduction.

The Production of Fertility in the First World

Infertility is not a deficiency disease. As traumatic as the absence of children may be for some people, infertility is no more a disease than is the absence of other physical capabilities. Disability rights activists have long pointed out that physical handicaps should not be treated as diseases. Yet people continue to act as if infertility is a disease, encouraged by a technoscience that treats it as such by medicalizing infertility at primary cost to women.

What disease is being treated when most of the women leave IVF programs as infertile as when they arrived and, often, much more ravaged than when they came?[2] Furthermore, some of the women suffer from a rather unusual "disease": sterility that exists in another person, a male partner. They are unable to become pregnant because their *partners'* sperm is low in quantity and motility. There is no medical indication that *they* need treatment, yet they—not their male partners—undergo the in vitro fertilization procedures. This all happens so that his sparse and sluggish sperm can mate with her harvested eggs in the petri dish, only to be surgically implanted later on in her uterus.

Doctors increasingly expand the definition of infertility. The currently accepted medical definition is inability to conceive after one year of intercourse without contraception.[3]

In the last decade, the number of years has dwindled from two to one. However, as many as half the couples seeking treatment for infertility will conceive in the usual heterosexual way, without any help from fertility treatments, and even after technical fertility treatment has failed.[4]

Infertility is not sterility. Infertility may be temporary, whereas sterility is permanent infertility. The accepted definition of infertility fails to take into account the fact that, for older women and those who have recently stopped using oral contraceptives, conceiving is likely to take longer than one year. The definition conflates inability to conceive with difficulty in conceiving quickly. This creates anxiety and concern for many couples and routes a large number of women into unnecessary and experimental medical treatment.

News stories that wrongly quote infertility statistics add to the confusion and anxiety. It has been widely reported that one out of six or seven U.S. couples is infertile and that infertility is on the rise due to the spread of sexually transmitted diseases and women who delay childbearing. Frequently cited are three National Surveys conducted by the National Center for Health Statistics (NCHS) in 1965, 1976, and 1982. According to NCHS statistician William Mosher, however, these statistics have been misinterpreted. The correct figure is one in twelve couples is infertile. Neither the percentage nor the actual number of infertile couples increased between 1965 and 1982.[5]

Yet one still hears about an epidemic of infertility.[6] In the same way that the definition of infertility has been expanded, infertility specialists claim that the number of people who are infertile has expanded exponentially during the last decade. In 1988, however, the Office of

Technology Assessment report on infertility confirmed that "there has been no increase in either the number of infertile couples or the overall incidence of infertility in the population."[7] What has increased is the number of fertility specialists and thus the corresponding number of office visits to physicians for infertility services (from 600,000 in 1968 to 1.6 million in 1984). If there is no real increase in the number of infertile couples or in the overall percentage of infertility in the population, fertility specialists still have been very adept at drumming up business. Medicine is hyping infertility to market technological reproduction.

The courts have also tried to expand the definition of infertility in cases of contractual reproduction. In the first 1987 Baby M trial, which took place in New Jersey Superior Court, Judge Sorkow went to great lengths to define infertility in the broadest way possible. During the trial, it was learned that Dr. Betsy Stern, the wife of litigant Bill Stern, father of the baby, had a mild form of multiple sclerosis. She was not technically infertile, even by the broad standards of the accepted definition of infertility, since this disability does not render women unable to conceive or carry to term. Doctors are divided on what risks a pregnancy would entail for women with such a mild form of multiple sclerosis, but the court held that "a risk, though minimal, remains a risk to one who is faced with it and so it was a genuine risk to Mrs. Stern."[8] The court then took this notion of risk and defined infertility as "something more than ability [sic] to conceive. 'Infertility' as applied in this case shall mean the inability to conceive and carry to term without serious threat of harm to one's physical well-being."[9] Thus the range of infertility was inflated by the courts, as it has been by the medical profession.

It is not infertility, but the medical and professional production of infertility, that is expanding. Physicians give meaning to the term and define it in their own interests, especially since the advent of new reproductive technologies. Infertility is being produced to enable technological reproduction; the technologies are not being produced to enable the infertile. If a couple is defined as infertile after only one year rather than two or three, the woman all the more quickly becomes a candidate for technological treatment. Such supposed infertility is the result of impatience rather than inability to conceive. Many couples do want quick answers and quick solutions, and reproductive technologists are quick to provide the appearance of both, but appearances are deceiving.

Although the definition of infertility is expanding, the portrait of the infertile is shrinking to a deceptively homogenous image. Being generated is a public picture of the typical infertile woman as a woman who never has been able to conceive, who is desperate for children, and who is clamoring for reproductive technologies. In fact, many women and their male partners who use technological reproduction have not always been infertile. Many have had children in the past, perhaps in a previous marriage, but want children in a subsequent marriage. In a large percentage of those undergoing IVF treatment, for example, either the woman or her partner has had children in a prior relationship, yet IVF is often thought of as a treatment only for the forever infertile. Many couples also have had children in their present marriage, at an earlier point, but later the woman cannot conceive again due to either male- or female-factor reasons, so she becomes a candidate for technological reproduction.

Infertile women especially are portrayed as desperate for children. One woman, in responding to an article in *Ms.* magazine, related that the classic comment whenever anyone discovers she is infertile is, "'Have you thought about adoption (or in vitro, or surrogacy)' as though simply getting a child somehow will solve the problem. It is assumed that in order to be a whole family, we must desire and seek to obtain a child."[10] In choosing to live without children, this woman appears abnormal to others, especially people with children. Her privacy is frequently invaded when people persist in asking why she has no children. ("Don't they like kids?" "Are they prejudiced against children who aren't related genetically?") Or people relate countless stories about friends and relatives who adopted and love their child as if she or he were "their own." The letter writer concludes that there would be fewer ethical dilemmas created by the use of reproductive technologies if people accepted infertility and did not pressure the infertile to have a child at any cost.

There is also a homogenous understanding of groups who support and advocate for the infertile. Not all these groups promote the use of reproductive technologies. For example, some self-help groups for women with infertility problems formed with the express purpose of avoiding the abuse of technological reproduction and examining the meaning of infertility and its solutions.[11] The more well known and better financed, however, are groups like RESOLVE, a clearinghouse of information and a support network for the infertile that provides referrals to in vitro fertilization programs.

Finally, the public image of the infertile is uniformly female. Male-factor infertility, however, is as common as female-factor. In cases where infertility can be causally explained and linked with sex, about half the number of infertile couples cannot have children because of problems associated with the man's infertility.[12] In reality, about one-third of all cases of infertility are due to female-factor problems; about one-third to male-factor problems; and the remaining third are unexplained cases (idiopathic infertility).[13] In spite of what is known about the equal occurrence of male infertility, often in infertility assessments the male partner is not tested or is tested only after the woman has undergone extensive and exhaustive evaluation. And frequently, men refuse to undergo such tests, viewing them as offensive to their virility.

Between 23 and 60 percent of women undergo IVF treatment because of their male partners' infertility.[14] Because women undergo the procedures, many men do not have to acknowledge their infertility. Women bear the burden of being perceived as the deficient person in need of repair, as well as the risks of the procedures. Like the women whose male partners want to hire surrogates to carry "their" children, the wives of men who are infertile allow the procedure to go forward, bearing the responsibility for their husbands.

The causes of male infertility, like the causes of female infertility, have been widely debated. There is tentative agreement on the following factors: The most common causes of male infertility are inability to ejaculate sperm or sluggish sperm motility (movement) ranging from 4 to 0 on the infertility scale, that is, from slow swimming to no swimming sperm. Low or no sperm motility is caused by hormone deficiencies and blockages in the genital vessels and by specific genital tract infections, which may result from venereal diseases. Other factors, such as the influence of environmental or workplace pollutants, may in turn affect sperm motility. Sperm that may be contaminated from pollution can also produce reactions in female partners, such as antibodies that respond to the toxins in the sperm or allergic reactions that alter the chemistry of the womb in ways that are detrimental to the developing embryo. As environmentalist John Elkington put it, "The sperm may yet prove to be the Trojan Horse of reproductive toxicology."[15] It is the egg, however, that is the workhorse of technological reproduction.

The causes of infertility in women have been more widely discussed, although little money and research specifically devoted to preventing infertility have been forthcoming. The most commonly cited causes of female-factor infertility are blocked fallopian tubes or tubal disease; pelvic inflammatory disease (PID) caused by, among other things, past use of an IUD; past iatrogenic (doctor-induced) "diseases" such as adhesions or occlusion resulting from gynecological surgery, C-sections, and abortions; sexually transmitted diseases (STDs), the most common of which is chlamydia, that can damage the female reproductive system; ovulatory dysfunction; and endometriosis.

In 1985, doctors in Australia, the then-IVF capital of the world, decried the amount of money and resources being funneled into IVF research and treatment, money they alleged could be better spent on infertility prevention. One doctor argued, "The unsolved problem of pelvic inflammatory disease, occurring in apparently younger and younger age groups, is hardly answered appropriately by more and more costly emphasis on the exciting treatment of infertility by microsurgery to fallopian tubes and by IVF programs."[16] In Victoria, the 1985 budget allocated 25,000 Australian dollars for STD research and prevention; meanwhile, the state financed one million dollars of IVF expenditures. Critics argued that all the money and attention going into IVF should be diverted to STD clinics.

Instead, in all countries with IVF programs, money and research have been funneled into variations of the in vitro fertilization procedure. As the production of infertility initially led to the production of in vitro fertilization, IVF has produced its own technological progeny.

The Technological Parent of Them All

In vitro fertilization is "the site at which all [new reproductive] practices converge and move outward in an ever-expanding chain reaction of uncertain effects."[17] It is also the technique that has captured the most media attention. Fifteen or twenty years ago, IVF was seen as a fringe technology. Today it is regarded as the most conservative of the new reproductive technologies and used as a venue for all the others. Lawrence Sucsy, whose firm invests in medical technologies, told a reporter that he decided to invest in embryo transfer research and technology after reading a poll showing that 75 percent of the women interviewed approved of IVF. "That convinced me that women would also accept embryo transfer, so I threw myself on the railroad track.[!]"[18]

In the United States today, over 200 institutions perform IVF treatment.[19] In the absence of federal funds for research on in vitro fertilization, the tab has been picked up by patients, pharmaceutical companies, universities and hospitals, and private organizations often relying on venture capital. A large number of these centers are for-profit "fertility institutes." Although rates vary, a conservative figure that clients pay is about 4,000 to 7,000 dollars per IVF cycle.[20] Many women return for two, five, and some for more than ten cycles.

The United States, however, is not the reproductive technology capital of the world. France and Australia compete for this title. For example, France has more IVF centers per capita than any other country in the world; Australia has had the highest success rates and an infusion of government spending for the technologies. Australia has exported its IVF technology to the United States and other countries. This venture, first launched as IVF Australia and now called IVF America, has established many for-profit fertility centers in this country, as well as in Europe and many developing countries.[21] It is also the first IVF company in the United States to go public with a stock offering (Nasdaq Small Cap) in June 1992, which, it hopes, will provide the capital for IVF America to become "the first provider of fertility services with clinics blanketing the country."[22] In 1990, however, the Federal Trade Commission had faulted IVF America for advertisements and brochures that mislead clients about their chance of taking home a baby. In April of that same year, the company signed a consent decree with the commission promising to be more forthright with customers, but as recently as April 1992, the Federal Trade Commission stated that IVF America had failed to comply with the decree by continuing to promote misleading advertising about its success rates.[23]

Despite the absence of federal support in the United States, the technological reproduction market is expanding rapidly. Groups of doctors have joined the entrepreneurial fray and have helped spawn a rapid proliferation of new drugs and technologies. For example, two doctors own Pacific Fertility Medical Centers, a chain of seven IVF clinics, which eventually could be a multiple billion dollar annual business.[24] In its 1989 IVF-ET Registry, the American Fertility Society, obviously concerned about the proliferation of IVF centers and their potential to compromise the success statistics of the more quality-controlled clinics, concluded, "It would be a very unfortunate trend if the number of IVF clinics continues to increase enough to compromise volume per clinic and counterbalance the positive effects of experience. These factors undoubtedly obscure the progressive improvement of results from year to year in well-established programs."[25]

As with IVF America, the success rates have not been outstanding, even in well-established programs. In fact, rarely has a technology that has had such dismal success rates been so quickly accepted. In the early 1980s, newspapers and scientific journal articles reported IVF success rates of 25 to 30 percent. Typical of such reports was an article in *Ob. Gyn. News,* a publication with a high physician subscription base. "The success rate for in-vitro fertilization decreases as maternal age increases, ranging from 30 percent among women in their twenties to 6 percent for women over age 40."[26] In these early articles, doctors faulted aging women for lower success rates, but there was no blame attributed to the techniques themselves or to unsuccessful clinics. And no mention was made of the statistical ways in which success was misrepresented by the IVF centers.

In 1985, journalists Gena Corea and Susan Ince undertook a comprehensive study of hospitals and centers offering IVF services. Their report, first published in the *Medical Tribune* and since reprinted elsewhere, stated that clinics varied in the way they reported their success statistics. Definitions of pregnancy varied widely (You thought you knew one when you saw one, but not in the realm of IVF statistics). Clinics often measured success rates not by the number of live births but by the number of successful implantations that never resulted in births or even by the number of chemical pregnancies (elevation of

hormone level that may but often does not result in an ongoing pregnancy. IVF America obscured its success rates in these ways.) Half of
the clinics in the study had never had a single live birth. Even some of
the IVF experts admitted that "it's easy to fudge results. People can say
they have a 50 percent success rate and there's no way to check that,"
admitted Alan De Cherney of Yale University.[27] Dr. John Biggers,
another IVF expert, acknowledged as early as 1981 that the probability
of getting a live birth once a woman has been selected for egg recovery
is "extremely small."[28] And as biologist Renate Klein has observed,
"The success rates do not go up: if anything, they come tumbling down
because of the increasing supervision . . . as [IVF clinics] are asked to
report their figures to government committees. . . ."[29]

Often clinics report success rates "per transfer." Women who try
again and again for babies during the in vitro process undergo multiple
transfers (implants) of fertilized eggs from the petri dish to their
wombs. Per-transfer rates, however, do not tell us the number of children per mother. Because women who take fertility drugs often become pregnant with multiple embryos and deliver twins, triplets, and
even quadruplets, reporting the number of babies per transfer gives the
impression of one child per mother. Additionally, most clinics, regardless of their methods of reporting success, do not include the number
of women who drop out of IVF programs because they cannot produce
eggs, even with the use of fertility drugs, or those whose eggs cannot
be fertilized. These women, of whom there are many, would lower the
success rates much more than they are now, and thus they are not
counted in the statistics.[30]

U.S. newspapers continued to report success rates for IVF varying
from 10 to 30 percent even after the Corea-Ince study was published.
Clinicians contended that the Corea-Ince study was outdated and represented only the early phases of IVF treatment. However, in 1988 the
U.S. Office of Technology Assessment (OTA) confirmed the dismal
findings.[31] Still, it was not until the Wyden congressional subcommittee published its national survey of U.S. IVF clinics in March 1989 that
a minimal acknowledgment of these low rates appeared in the press.
The Wyden national survey reported a "take-home baby" rate of 9 percent, but it noted that many clinics base success on rates of clinical
pregnancy per attempted egg recovery methods rather than on live

births.[32] In the late 1980s, England's take-home baby rate was 8.6 percent; France's 6.9 percent; and Australia's 8.8 percent, decreasing to 4.8 percent for a healthy child.[33]

The number of *healthy* children born is also hidden in the IVF success statistics. Live or "take-home" baby rates do not necessarily mean unproblematic births. A 1987 Australian perinatal report noted the increased number of premature births—and thus of low weight babies in need of additional neonatal care—associated with IVF (26.9 percent for 1985).[34] The same study reported that the mortality rate of children for the first twenty-eight days after birth was 47.5 deaths for every 1,000 births, which is about four times higher than the normal rate of 12.2 deaths per 1,000 births. The perinatal report also documented that congenital abnormalities among IVF babies were greater than expected. Two types of congenital malformations were reported: spina bifida (5 times the expected rate); and a serious heart defect called transposition of the great vessels (6.7 times the expected rate).[35] A British report chronicled the high proportion of multiple births in 1987 (24 percent) due to superovulation and multiple implants.[36] For multiple-birth babies, the incidence of premature birth, low birth weight, and postnatal deaths is far worse than for single births.[37] These figures have been confirmed from other IVF clinics around the world, when those clinics are made accountable for reporting them through governmental monitoring.

In addition, the Australian perinatal report noted other difficulties associated with IVF treatment: the risk of pregnancies occurring outside the uterus, and of ectopic pregnancies in particular, is five times greater than normal; the risk of miscarriage in IVF is two to three times higher than normal; and 43.9 percent of deliveries are done by cesarian section compared to 15 to 18 percent (25 percent in the U.S.) in natural deliveries.[38]

Virtually no studies have been done in the United States documenting similar problems of low birth weight, premature births, the risk of pregnancies conceived outside the uterus, the rate of miscarriage, and congenital abnormalities. A 1989 U.S. study done by Dr. James Mills, a researcher at the National Institute of Child Health and Human Development, appeared in *The Journal of Pediatrics*. This study compared eighty-three babies conceived by IVF with ninety-three babies conceived normally and found no increased risk of abnormal development. However, the babies were all conceived at one center, the Norfolk Clinic in Virginia, and did show an increase of abnormalities (two IVF infants had major malformations compared to one in the normal group). This was reported as "statistically insignificant," with some newspaper headlines describing Mills's study as "reassuring,"[39] and others as "dispelling fears of high rate of birth defects."[40] Given the small numbers of children involved and the restriction of the study to one clinic, however, this study cannot be compared to the numbers of cases and the long-term statistics documented in the Australian perinatal study that was conducted over a six-year time span and reported on 1,700 live births. Unfortunately, there are no federal and hardly any state monitoring and regulatory mechanisms in the United States for overseeing any part of the IVF process—number of children born, number of birth abnormalities, and, least likely, numbers of women damaged by any aspect of the IVF treatment. In the absence of such monitoring and regulation, the American Fertility Society, whose membership is largely composed of clinicians and researchers involved with these technologies, claims to monitor itself (see chapter 4).

The problems and the lack of success of IVF treatment have, ironically, become the accepted justification for developing new technical variations of the IVF procedure such as GIFT, ZIFT, and TUDOR.[41] Earlier, scientists argued for the addition of superovulation—medical sorties of powerful fertility drugs used to blast the ovaries into multiple egg production—to the IVF regimen. In kindler and gentler terminology, blasting the ovaries is referred to as "stimulating ovulation," thus enabling clinicians to "capture" eggs not accessible to laparoscopy. But these techniques have brought with them their own specific problems.[42]

Dangerous fertility drugs, such as Clomid and Pergonal, have been administered not only in concert with IVF but also as a solo treatment to stimulate multiple eggs in women having difficulty conceiving. The most publicized instance of fertility drugs gone wrong was the U.S. birth of the Frustaci septuplets. Although they were not born of an IVF procedure, their births illustrate the particular problems that result when women are placed on fertility drugs. Four of the septuplets died within four months after their birth in May of 1985, and the remaining three lingered on with continuing medical problems, attached to monitors so that their mother could shout at them when they "forgot" to breathe. At age five they still had heart and eye problems, suffered lifelong disabilities including cerebral palsy and severe developmental difficulties, and Mrs. Frustaci has a kidney problem. The Frustacis sued the clinic, the oldest fertility center in Los Angeles, and the fertility specialist for malpractice, for the high dosage of Pergonal that Mrs. Frustaci was given, and for the doctor's alleged negligence to monitor the number of follicles by ultrasound. In 1990, the Frustacis settled their suit for six million dollars.[43]

Since these same fertility drugs are now used on women in IVF treatment, researchers have begun to investigate their use in IVF programs. In a ground-breaking and extensive study of fertility drugs, particularly of clomiphene citrate (commercial name, Clomid), Renate Klein and Robyn Rowland document the list of deleterious effects associated with Clomid's administration. In addition to causing hyperstimulation of the ovaries and cysts, clomiphene is cited in numbers of scientific studies in conjunction with an increased incidence of cancer in women. Since fertility drugs cause rapid cell growth, this is not surprising, and the possibility of a cancer epidemic among women on infertility programs looms large.[44] Thus in January 1993 the U.S. Food and Drug Administration (FDA) required makers of certain fertility drugs to add information to their labels on the possible link between the drugs and ovarian cancer. Specifically cited were Pergonal and Serophene (Serono Laboratories) and Clomiphene Citrate (Marian Merrell Dow).[45]

Klein and Rowland note also the similarities between DES and clomiphene, raising the question about long-term effects in women who take the drug and in their children. Research reports in the 1980s have further highlighted chromosomal abnormalities in human egg cells produced by clomiphene induction and also the risk of congenital malformation, which increases by a factor of two.[46] Increasingly, clomiphene is used in what some refer to as "hormonal cocktails" (that is, a combination of drugs), because it alone does not produce enough mature eggs. These "hormonal cocktails" only increase the dangers to women who are given the drug in IVF programs.

With the continuing use of fertility drugs and multiple implants during the IVF process, the medical need for new technologies to solve the problems caused by these very drugs and implants (for example, multiple pregnancies) expands. Fetal reduction (see chapter 3), for example, is used to selectively terminate a certain number of fetuses in women who become multiply pregnant as a result of fertility drugs and/or multiple implants. Doctors inject a saline solution into the uterus to abort some of the fetuses, a procedure that can cause bleeding, infections, danger of premature labor, and even the loss of all fetuses. There is concern also about damage to any fetuses that remain after others are "reduced." Yet Western faith in medical progress has reached the point where people accept, without criticism, that past technological problems need more technological solutions, which can themselves turn into problems. This is the height of technological determinism, and women are left with an increased dependency on more and more questionable technical solutions.

In other areas of medical treatment, technologies that are laden with as many problems as new reproductive technologies, such as experimental AIDS drugs and cancer chemotherapy, are used only in life-threatening cases. For many Western women, the inability to conceive after a period of one year—now called infertility—is treated with extreme procedures as though it is a life-threatening illness. In the East and in the developing South, however, it is the ability to conceive "too many" children—fertility—that has been portrayed as a life-threatening disease to women, nations, and the environment.

The Case of Norplant

Third World countries have long served as testing grounds for contraceptives, a fact finally recognized in a report of the International Social Science Council and UNESCO. At their 1985 conference, these UN groups referred specifically to Third World peoples at risk of exploitation as test populations for biomedical products or used as secondary markets where developed countries unload products no longer legal or in demand in their own nations.

The 1985 UN document also recognized that those most at risk from the new reproductive technologies are women and that women who are poor, migrant, refugee, of an ethnically different minority, and who speak a different language may be at particular risk. Disadvantaged women in the so-called First World who have little access to health care are also at higher risk of illness and disability and of not being informed of potential hazards of biomedical procedures.[47]

Medical exploitation of poor women, particularly in the Third World, has been historically widespread. The pill was initially tested on women in Puerto Rico. Women in the Third World have been given stronger doses of hormones in three-month contraceptive injections and pills because undernourished bodies store fewer hormones and secrete them more quickly. Many women in these countries still have the Dalkon Shield implanted, an IUD taken off the market in the United States.[48] In fact, after A. H. Robins was forced to halt U.S. retail sales of the Dalkon Shield in 1974, it retrieved unmarketed shields and sold 697,000 of them to USAID (United States Agency for International Development) for distribution in the Third World through the International Planned Parenthood Federation, the Pathfinder Fund, the Population Council, and Family Planning International Assistance.[49] Women in developing countries have also been the primary experimental population for multicenter[50] testing of contraceptive implants, injectables, and antipregnancy vaccines. This has been the case with Norplant, the long-acting contraceptive, which is surgically implanted.

Norplant is a synthetic hormone called progestin that inhibits ovulation. It is implanted just under the skin of a woman's arm and released at a slow, supposedly even, rate into her body over a five-year period. Norplant has been one of the favorite contraceptives of the international population and family planning establishment, initially researched and developed by one of their own, the Population Council. It is now marketed in the United States by Wyeth-Ayerst of Philadelphia, but the Population Council receives 4 percent of the company's profits.[51]

One of the initial test sites for Norplant was Brazil. At the time that the testing of Norplant was initiated on Brazilian women, the military dictatorship was still in power, and there was effectively no public input into the decision. The government presented testing as a *fait accompli* that would involve seven clinics and a total of two thousand women. The tests performed were called "preintroductory tests." Dr. Ana Regina Gomes Dos Reis, senior official in the Brazilian Ministry of Health, which later investigated the outcome of the Norplant testing, clarified a key difference between tests that are actual trials and so-called preintroductory tests.

In the 1984 annual report of the Population Council . . . tests like this were called pre-introductory. In other words, the tests do not concern so much detailed analysis of each reaction of the woman to a new drug, but rather concern forming strategies for establishing the method, encouraging it to be accepted by women, and motivating doctors and nurses to recommend it. They are tests that use marketing techniques rather than clinical and epidemiological ones.[52]

In 1985, when there was a more democratic climate in Brazil, feminist groups helped activate a government committee study of Norplant. The committee investigated the irregularities, contradictions, and methodological errors of the entire Norplant testing in Brazil but, most importantly, interviewed women who had received the implants. Committee members, including feminists and congresswomen, found that Norplant spawned many complications: dramatic change in body weight; heavy bleeding and menstrual irregularities; and severe alterations of the central nervous system, among others.[53]

For the Population Council, however, the reported complications were simply "cause for removal." In the medical literature, these removals are recorded as "woman requested removal," or "woman did not complete the trials," rather than "clinical complications made removal necessary." Thus the removals do not become part of the statistical ledger of serious complications compromising the distribution of the drug in other countries. In 1986 the Brazilian government canceled its authorization for the Norplant trials. Today, with a new government and a new Ministry of Health, the case for Norplant has been reopened.

For women in Bangladesh, Norplant testing was set to begin in 1981. "From the beginning, Norplant was promoted to the Government of Bangladesh as *more effective than sterilization*."[54] The Bangladesh Fertility Research Program (BFRP), the national family planning and biomedical research organization in Bangladesh, placed an ad in the country's newspapers billing Norplant as "a wonderful innovation of modern science" but not disclosing that the implant was still in its experimental stage.

In October 1981 Farida Akhter, executive director of UBINIG, a Bangladeshi group that as part of its ongoing work monitors population control measures, wrote an article in one of the same newspapers where the above ad had been placed, raising questions and criticizing the lack of ethics and the unproven claims connected with the implant's proposed launch. Interestingly, the first sentence of the BFRP ad had made clear, "This method is for women." Akhter underscored that the promoters made a point of emphasizing gender "to make Norplant acceptable to the people and the government because exclusion of men makes the method politically safe."[55] Following a protest initiated by UBINIG, the tests were postponed but relaunched in 1985. Promoters made no mention of the earlier advertisement in 1981.

As in Brazil, it became clear that the Bangladeshi BFRP's 1985 objectives in launching the implant were to *promote* it, not to look into its safety aspects. "The objective of the research was to create the conditions for the *mass promotion* of Norplant within the family planning programme of Bangladesh. Interestingly, this is also the explicit objective of the Population Council."[56] Furthermore, UBINIG reported that the second round of Bangladeshi research and testing of Norplant in 1985 was initiated in very secretive fashion and not well publicized.

False and misleading information was given to women clients at the hospitals and clinics dispensing the implant. None were told that the drug was experimental, that animal testing had not been completed, or that the implant could cause complications. Among the claims were that the drug was 100 percent effective (it has a 3 percent failure rate); that women themselves can remove the implant when they want (this is dangerous); and that after removal, fertility returns within a year (unproven). When the BFRP made an initial report to a conference in Bangladesh in 1986, the director admitted that of the 600 women who were given Norplant in 1985 and 1986, only 187, that is, 31 percent, continued on the method after 1986. Over half, 56 percent of the women, reported changes in their menstrual pattern.[57]

In December 1985 UBINIG began to interview women who had been put on the contraceptive. "Because the Norplant study had been conducted silently—if not secretly—we received no cooperation from the medical centers who took part in the trial when we asked to speak to women who had the Norplant capsules implanted."[58] Of the ten women they managed to find who had started using Norplant in one village of Basila, three had stopped using it within the year, some resorting to removal of the implant themselves. All ten had experienced health problems since beginning Norplant: amenorrhea, loss of appetite, vertigo, burning sensations in hands and feet, general body aches and weakness, and leukorrhea (a potentially serious vaginal infection). UBINIG reports, however, that within the BFRP

> the follow-up monitoring was done to record medical problems of interest to the research project but with little care for the safety of the clients. We found that amenorrhea was a very frequent problem—all 10 women in our study suffered from it—but the tendency of the centres was to trivialize this problem and even to justify it as the price to pay for birth control. The women had to plead for the removal of the capsules, sometimes go to the centre two or three times. In this way, one could argue, more research results were accumulated: further evidence, we believe, for the unethical conduct of the trial.[59]

On November 6, 1986, UBINIG called a press conference on the Norplant trials in Bangladesh and asked the government to halt the research of the BFRP. All the dailies carried UBINIG's findings and expressed concern about the unethical nature of the research: the lack of informed consent, the withholding of relevant information to clients, and the nondisclosure of complications. Neither the BFRP nor the government responded, and at this writing the experiment continues. UBINIG continues to protest the Norplant trials citing their unethical experimentation on poor, vulnerable women who are used as guinea pigs for international contraceptive research and who are the recipients of an unsafe contraceptive method being used for population control.

In 1990, UBINIG joined with FINRRAGE, an international feminist network operating in more than 35 countries that monitors the development of reproductive and genetic technologies and their effects on women worldwide, in organizing and hosting the first international conference to be held in a developing country on reproductive technologies and genetic engineering. One hundred and five attendees, the majority from Asian countries, took part. Also in attendance were many Bangladeshi journalists who, prior to the meeting, had not heard much that was critical about population control, harmful contraceptives, and their influence on women's health. The Comilla Declaration, which emerged from this international meeting, condemned Norplant,

Depo-Provera, Net-en, and antifertility vaccines, among other drugs, and called for a regional campaign against these methods of population control.[60]

Also in 1990, the Sixth International Women's Health Congress, held in the Philippines, drafted a resolution opposed to the testing, research, and development of Norplant, antipregnancy vaccines, and the new chemical abortifacient, RU 486. It stated,

> Norplant, a long acting hormonal contraceptive, developed and promoted by the Population Council, has been introduced in many countries of the world, particularly in those countries which have coercive population control programmes. Through experiences and research it has been established that the six-capsule implant (Norplant) is harmful, has potential long-term risks for women and children they bear, and that it takes control of our fertility out of our hands.[61]

Norplant is the most recent in a long line of contraceptives that, along with sterilization, are viewed as technical solutions to women's fertility that is supposedly out of control. Most of these drugs and technologies have been launched by Western population organizations in conjunction with the governments of developing countries and related research agencies, such as the BFRP in Bangladesh.

Recently, population control groups have also begun to make alliances with various women's health activists and organizations. The cooperation between feminists and the population planning establishment signals a disturbing trend as these alliances increasingly provide population planners with the learning and language to rationalize, not change, their population control policies and practices. At the Sixth International Women's Health Meeting held in the Philippines, reproductive health consultant Marge Berer called upon women's health activists to strive for influence within the population planning organizations to develop a feminist population policy.[62] UBINIG director, Farida Akhter, and other women from developing countries rejected this approach, stating that the notion of a "feminist population policy" is as ridiculous and oppressive as a "feminist policy on exploitation," a "feminist policy of racism or race purification," and a "feminist policy on war." A so-called feminist population policy, they pointed out, is nothing but an "innovative strategy of the population controllers to coopt feminists to implement population control."[63]

Increasingly, population planners are meeting with feminist groups to implement strategies and enlist their support. For example, the Summer 1990 issue of *ISIS* Women's Health Journal, a publication of the Latin American and Caribbean Women's Health Network, carried an adulatory article on a meeting between women's health activists, feminists, and family planning groups hosted by the New York–based Population Council and numerous Mexican health and family planning organizations in Queretaro, Mexico. In the words of Amparo Claro, coordinator of the Latin American and Caribbean Women's Health Network, the meeting was motivated by the belief among population and family planning agencies that "given the poor track record of top-down policies and the maturity of the women's health movement, 'it is better, and more effective, to have women and feminists as friends than enemies.'"[64] The article in *ISIS* was subtitled, "Planners Face Up to Feminists in Family Planning Conference." Contrary to the confrontational spirit of its title, however, the *ISIS* article conveyed a sense of premature cooperation and gratitude for the "'historic and ground-breaking' . . . acceptance by policy-makers and funding agencies of feminist input into family planning programs."[65]

An article in the same issue of *ISIS* by Jose Barzelatto from the Ford Foundation launched the newspeak term for family planning, *reproductive health*. Barzelatto betrays that population planners are capable of assimilating the language of feminism, which they then use to bolster, not change, their practices. Here lies the basic problem inherent in the collaboration between population planners and feminists/women's health activists.

The goal of allying feminist groups and population planning organizations is fraught with the danger that feminists will be swept along by the greater power, economic resources, and reputation of the family planning establishment, as national research groups have been in the past (for example, the BFRP in Bangladesh). The promotion of RU 486 in the United States has demonstrated that women's groups have joined more with population planning groups than the population groups with feminists. Many U.S. feminist organizations are promoting the chemical abortifacient or are remaining uncharacteristically neutral, with the result that the historically critical edge and the political viewpoint of the women's health movement have been muted. Nor have women's groups insisted that in-depth, independent, and nonaligned studies be done on the health and safety effects of the drug, beyond those reported by the drug's medical researchers and promoters.[66] Given the track record of the population establishment in promoting drugs and devices that have been dehumanizing and destructive to women, it appears that any alliance can only favor the goals of the population planners, goals that can be justifiably challenged as not in women's best interests.

Women as Population Polluters: Sex Predetermination Methods

Population planning has had the most drastic consequences in countries where sex predetermination technologies have been promoted and used to solve so-called population problems. When sex predetermination techniques were first discussed, initial focus was on a man-child pill. As Clare Booth Luce observed, "What theological objections could the pope himself raise to a birth-control method that simply permitted parents to choose a son in preference to a daughter? After all, God did."[67] Luce summed up the popular support for this man-child technology; John Postgate articulated the scientific rationale in 1973. Postgate, a molecular biologist at the University of Sussex in England, wrote in the *New Scientist* that the man-child pill should be promoted in developing countries especially because "among most African, Asian, Central and South American peoples, this prejudice [for having male children] amounts to an obsession."[68] And Paul Ehrlich, avatar of the population and environment movement, articulated the environmental rationale in his 1971 work called *The Population Bomb*: "If a simple method could be found to guarantee that first-born children were males, then population control measures in many areas would be somewhat eased."[69]

No pill has yet been developed to produce boy children. The term *man-child pill* has become an inclusive and popular term for various technologies that are now being developed to determine sex before birth or even before conception. Some methods, such as separating x- from y-bearing sperm before conception, are still in the experimental stage. A U.S. entrepreneur of sperm-separation technology, however, claims a 70 to 80 percent success rate with this method and has set up a chain of clinics in India, Jordan, Pakistan, Egypt, Malaysia, Singapore, and Taiwan, as well as in California (Gametrics, Inc.).[70] The most reliable sex predetermination technologies, however, are postconception methods of amniocentesis, chorionic villus sampling, ultrasound, and preimplantation diagnosis using a DNA probe to evaluate the embryo after an egg has been fertilized in the IVF process. IVF technology allows for the embryo to be tested in a petri dish for, among other things, its sex, before it is placed into the womb of a woman.

Partly for sex predetermination goals, IVF clinics have been established in some Third World countries—in Brazil, India, Malaysia, and Indonesia, for example. Clinics have been deluged with requests from financially well off women affected not only by infertility but by the stigma of not having produced a son by usual heterosexual means. For certain women, this means loss of respect, divorce, banishment, and sometimes death.

For scientists, however, the establishment of IVF centers in countries such as India offers enormous potential for research in the manipulation of both fertility and infertility and thus for population control. One researcher, Dr. Anand Kumar, the director of the Institute for Research in Reproduction in Bombay, stated in an interview that "an understanding of [IVF-Embryo Transfer] may provide clues as to how to *induce infertility in fertile couples* as a means of family planning."[71]

Many of these IVF clinics have been engineered by Western scientists and entrepreneurs but staffed with local doctors. They are seen as a commercial boon in a situation where neither the market nor the research possibilities are hampered by the few restrictions placed on IVF centers in Western contexts. The exporting of IVF and related technologies by companies such as PIVET Australia[72] to Hong Kong and Malaysia, for example, has expanded exponentially the technical possibilities for manipulation of fertility and infertility in the developing world.

In India's population control programs, for example, female feticide after amniocentesis has been called the most ideal and rational solution to the population explosion.[73] Population planners in India have generated a net reproduction rate (NRR) target, stipulating an ideal of one woman replacing her mother. At the same time, woman are encouraged to have two or three births, meaning that the "excess" number of females that could be born must be terminated at the fetal stage to maintain the NRR of one. Census data reveals a dramatic skewing of sex ratios to the extent that for every 1,000 men, there are now only 920 women in India.[74] In some states, such as Haryan, there are only 874 females for every 1,000 males, the lowest ratio of any of India's fourteen major states.[75]

The situation is so serious that the United Nations Children's Fund, in a report prepared for the Indian government that has not been released, found that preference for male children is blatant in the wide and cheap availability of sex predetermination technologies, even in rural areas, and that girls get less medical attention, are neglected, fed last, malnourished, and in some cases starved to death.[76] This situation has led many to begin speaking about the world's "missing women." According to Harvard economist Amartya Sen, over 100 million women are "missing" worldwide, and the situation is worst in the Asian countries, particularly China and India.[77]

Sex predetermination mania, however, is not mainly the preoccupation of people in Third World countries. In the West, research tells us what we already know—that the preference for male children is rampant, especially for firstborns, and people's next-ranked expressed preference is not for girl children but for "either."[78] Often amniocentesis or other tests are done, purportedly for reasons such as genetic screening, so that parents do not have to disclose their desire to know the sex of the fetus. In a liberal context where sex equality is the rhetorical norm, such reasons are kept private, as are abortions that often follow upon sex predetermination.

Given the more articulated preference for male children in many Third World countries, however, and the less restrictive environment in which these facilities are allowed to flourish, it is not surprising that almost 80,000 female fetuses have been aborted during a five-year period in India.[79] To many doctors, these sex predetermination tests are not a discriminatory and drastic way of achieving both population and male preference goals, because they say it is the women themselves who ask for the procedure. What the statistics and sex ratios do not tell us is that given the realities of female infanticide, female malnutrition, female prostitution, dowry, and the devaluation of daughters in general, it is not surprising that many women ask for sex predetermination screening when the alternatives are so bleak for themselves and their potential daughters. Less frequently mentioned is the pressure placed on women to submit to sex predetermination tests by husbands and relatives.[80] There is an enormous difference, however, in women succumbing to family and cultural pressure to produce boy children and doctors' use of cultural norms to defend what they are doing.

Doctors also state that discrimination is not at issue here "because women are exploited anyway."[81] More discrimination, even of such a gynocidal variety, is thus no more and no less than what already exists. Practitioners shrug off the charge of discrimination, citing the social-cultural realities, as if social systems such as dowry and devaluation of women are immutable but, worse, should be augmented rather than changed. Using these arguments, female feticide is medicalized and thus made to seem normal.

This kind of self-interested, opportunistic defense shows an absence of care about women. As Vibuti Patel of the Bombay Women's Centre and organizer of the Forum Against Prenatal Sex Determination and Preselection Techniques has said, "By this logic it is also better to kill poor people or Third World masses rather than to let them suffer in poverty and deprivation."[82] Patel's position is similar to that of many Indian feminist and health groups who have taken action against the sex determination tests. Their concern is with the increasing gynocide as well as the fact that many Indian women continue to be tested and undergo successive abortions until they conceive sons. In a country where 70 percent of women have persistent anemia,[83] repeated abortions are a health hazard of monumental proportions.

Long active in the campaign against female feticide in India, Patel also makes clear the underlying misogyny of the tests. "Now discrimination starts in the womb and the only way existing laws can be changed is by making the abuse of amniocentesis a national issue, the way we did with bride burning."[84]

The Forum Against Prenatal Sex Determination and Preselection Techniques, a coalition of women's groups, health activists, doctors, lawyers, and research groups, has done just that. The forum has organized workshops and public debates, conducted demonstrations outside sex predetermination clinics, and postered suburban trains countering the advertising by the clinics. In one instance, the forum organized a mother-daughter rally on Children's Day in 1986 that captured much media attention. The coalition has also proposed and promoted legislation to prohibit the use of amniocentesis for sex predetermination.

Largely due to the efforts of the forum, a new law has been passed in the state of Maharashtra, the capital of which is Bombay, banning any prenatal tests to determine the sex of the fetus. Known as the Maharashtra Regulation of Prenatal Diagnostic Techniques Act, the law does, however, permit prenatal testing on women over thirty-five years of age who have a medical or family history of genetic disease to determine whether these will occur in the fetus. The law also prescribes prison sentences and fines for doctors, patients, and their families if found in violation of the law by an "appropriate authority." Unfortunately, the law has many loopholes, and two major demands of the forum—that no private practitioner be allowed to engage in sex predetermination, and that in no instance should a woman undergoing the amniocentesis test be punished—were not included in the act.[85]

Not content with the final legislation, the forum has adopted a many-faceted campaign to change aspects of the law that are unfair to women. It is also working to ensure compliance by closing up the law's loopholes—monitoring the fourteen laboratories in the state that do the actual analysis, and setting up watchdog committees to oversee the law's implementation. The forum will continue the struggle to pass central legislation for all India. At the same time, it is committed to a wider campaign of consciousness-raising and the creation of all necessary conditions to ensure women's freedom.

Sympathy for the Infertile?

The Indian women's campaign against sex predetermination testing holds many hopeful lessons for Western feminists. Perhaps the most significant is that women must not be incriminated by the accusation that opposing the technologies means lacking sympathy for those who "must resort" to them. The Forum Against Sex Determination and Sex Preselection Techniques in India was repeatedly confronted with the charge that they lacked compassion for women who felt compelled to undergo amniocentesis—women who would be rejected by husbands and families, women who bore the weight of poverty, and women who faced the threat of death if they failed to produce male children. The Indian women's successful campaign demonstrates a more genuine sympathy that truly betters the lives of women by working to end institutionalized misogyny and thus the conditions that make it necessary for women to resort to thwarting the birth of potential daughters.

In the West, feminists who oppose technological reproduction are likewise accused of "no sympathy for the infertile." The Indian women's campaign, however, teaches us to focus sympathy in the right place. To encourage technological reproduction in the name of sympathy for the infertile is to sentimentalize medical violation. As journalist Ann Pappert has written, "I am a feminist, a journalist who writes frequently on medical and health issues, and a woman with a fertility problem. Like many other infertile women, I initially looked upon reproductive technology as a beneficial option for infertile women, but after spending a year researching and writing on these technologies I have come to regard them as a highly destructive science that not only offers little benefit to women, but causes great harm."[86]

Pappert is one of the increasing number of women with an infertility condition who are speaking out against reproductive technologies. She notes that technological reproduction puts a huge burden on women, greater than the original burden of infertility, because now women have even less of a chance to say no to childbearing. Women feel pressured to try technological reproduction simply because it exists. Concerned relatives and friends ask the inevitable question, "Have you tried IVF?" If not, then obviously she has *not* done all she can, and in Western patriarchal society, she *must* do all she can to remedy this supposedly unnatural condition of childlessness.

Pappert also notes that some feminists have been reluctant to publicly criticize new reproductive technologies because they fear they will be seen as attacking infertile women who use the technologies. "Thus we have the absurd situation where before these feminists criticize the NRTs [new reproductive technologies] they often feel compelled to explain that they are not attacking infertile women who use these technologies. When feminists, particularly feminist health activists, take this position they are giving implied support for the technology whether they realize it or not."[87] In other words, sympathy reduces to pity for infertile women. It has been the alleged medical agenda to support these technologies in the name of sympathy (pity) for the infertile. In reality, this kind of sympathy stereotypes infertile women as desperate, unstable, "emotional basket cases, whose obsessive desire for a child precludes any ability to contribute to the debate on these technologies."[88] Instead, Pappert stresses that feminists engage women with infertility conditions in opposing these technologies.

In addition to joining forces with infertile women, feminists must disidentify with these technologies and also with the more "moderate" position arguing that if the technologies are regulated and imbued with woman-caring principles (whatever those might be, and however this might occur), they might serve women better. Regulation supports and promotes technological reproduction and encourages more women to hand over their bodies for medical experimentation. Those who advocate the better regulation of IVF, embryo transfer, or surrogacy as the answer to the dilemma of infertility only serve to prolong the dilemma by prolonging and proliferating the problem (see chapter 6). Technological reproduction—even when it is more quality controlled—is a band-aid solution that creates more medical victims. It is the quintessential personal solution to a social problem.

When, in 1962, Rachel Carson published *Silent Spring,* her formidable critique of pesticides in agriculture, the chemical companies, many scientists, and the press accused her of having no sympathy for the 10,000 people who die daily from malnutrition and starvation. The theme in all these criticisms was that "a world without pesticides is doomed to pestilence and famine."[89] As with Carson's detractors, critics of the critics of technological reproduction are mostly the drug companies, the scientists, and the press. Their message is that some women need these technologies. What they do not say is that *all* women are put in jeopardy by technological reproduction: by the ways in which they degrade and abuse women's bodies; by their expansionism into the lives of not just the infertile but the fertile; by the potential they hold for genetic engineering and the manipulation of life; by the increased loss of reproductive self-determination imposed by reproductive technological proliferation; and by the ways in which they corrupt choice, altruism, and reproductive freedom.

Those who advocate technological reproduction, claiming sympathy for the infertile, fail to extend that same sympathy to the thousands of Third World women who are rendered strategically infertile by mass sterilization, contraceptives, and sex predetermination. It is a sympathy, based on an ideology of reproductive liberalism, that neutralizes the violation of women that is inherent in these technologies, while appearing to be sensitive to women. And it is a sympathy that supports medical profiteering, professional ambition, and clinical adventurism over the bodies of women. Such a sympathy serves mainly to strengthen a society in which these technologies are presented as one big supermarket of options but where, in fact, women, reproduction, and motherhood are continuously created in the image of man and medicine.

Maternal Environments and Ejaculatory Fathers: New Definitions of Motherhood and Fatherhood

Technological reproduction constructs new definitions of motherhood and fatherhood that permeate every aspect of new reproductive arrangements. As political scientist Somer Brodribb has written, "Maternity and paternity are being redefined, but not by women."[1]

Motherhood has been construed as an instinct, a biological bond with a child, or an unquestioned state of being that is the essence or pinnacle of female existence. Especially in the IVF context, clinicians take for granted that all women mother or wish they could. Motherhood is so widely accepted as the core aspect of a woman's existence that it brooks no criticism. Even feminists have been reluctant to question the supposed need to mother defended by proponents of technological reproduction, thereby acquiescing to the view that motherhood is like a biological motor driving itself to fulfillment no matter what the obstacles and the costs to women. For the more poetic, motherhood becomes an inspirational metaphor or symbol for the caring, nurturing, and sensitivity that women bring to a world that is ravaged by conflict. In the background of the discussion on the new reproductive technologies is the credo, usually unprofessed, that a real woman is a mother, or one who acts like a mother.

In this chapter I examine the largely unexamined role of how normative motherhood—that is, the cultural expectation that all women
should mother and the subsequent behavior that accompanies this expectation—pervades discussion of the new reproductive technologies.
Even the arguments that are framed in opposition to the new reproductive technologies are mired in the morass of how motherhood has been
constructed for women. In addition, these technologies deconstruct
motherhood in ways that deprive women of even the remnants of
mother-right. For example, when a woman signs a surrogate contract,
her motherhood is rendered null and void.

Another aim of this chapter is to examine the political power of a
new norm of fatherhood grounded in male gametes and genes—what I
have called *ejaculatory fatherhood*. New reproductive arrangements
give a technological boost to the prominence of paternity and to the
power of fathers' rights that are fast growing in other contexts, such
as child custody disputes and child sexual abuse cases. In such cases
fathers increasingly are given legal custody of children and mothers are
penalized, in some instances with indeterminate jail sentences, for trying to protect their children. In two widely publicized cases, Virginia
Lalonde in Boston and Dr. Elizabeth Morgan in Washington, D.C., were
both imprisoned for refusing to disclose the whereabouts of their
daughters to the courts and to their alleged paternal abusers. Lalonde's
exhusband was awarded custody of their daughter in 1991 after a
lengthy court battle. Morgan was finally given custody of her daughter
in New Zealand, where she fled after being released from prison. She
obtained from the New Zealand courts what she could not obtain in the
United States—a fair hearing and protection for her daughter.

The same shift in the definition of paternal rights and power is
occurring in reproductive conflicts. In surrogacy and frozen embryo disputes, the ejaculator is called a father from the very moment that his
sperm fertilizes an egg. By dint of fertile ejaculation per se, men are
becoming fathers before taking on any parental relationship. As the new
reproductive technologies become more and more a part of the medical
and legal landscapes, the focus is on fetuses and the new breed of
"ejaculatory fathers." Fatherhood, not motherhood, is empowered by
the new reproductive techniques.

In the initial debate over surrogate contracts in the United States,
liberal proponents claimed that banning surrogacy would take women

back to the days of biology as destiny, a destiny that has confined women to the realm of institutionalized motherhood. They argued that legalizing surrogacy would liberate women by debiologizing motherhood, separating the child bearer from the child rearer and enabling women to become mothers without going through pregnancy and birth. This was somehow seen as intrinsic to women's liberation.

On the other hand, opponents of surrogacy, especially from the religious and conservative spectrum, invoked a maternal instinct or maternal-infant bonding to argue against surrogate contracts. They argued that surrogate contracts destroy the natural bond of mother and child and thus undermine the biological family. Even among ex-surrogates like Mary Beth Whitehead who have dedicated themselves to fighting surrogacy, the language of maternal instinct and motherhood essentialism,[2] rather than the language of feminism, has constructed their opposition to surrogacy.

It is father essentialism, however, that prevails as political right. The first 1987 New Jersey Superior Court decision in the Baby M case, commonly referred to as the Sorkow decision, upheld the validity of the surrogate contract and awarded custody of the child to Bill Stern. Judge Sorkow based his decision, in part, on Bill Stern's right to "genetic fulfillment." Few criticized this reinforcement of male biological destiny, a destiny that has historically conferred rights and power on men. The institution of *father-right* increasingly reduces women to "alternative reproductive vehicles," "incubators," and "rented wombs," all phrases that have been used by the medical and legal progenitors of reproductive technologies and contracts. This resurgence of father-right is made invisible in judicial decisions that uphold the validity of surrogate contracts and in new legislation that permissively regulates such contracts.

The Spermatic Market: Surrogate Stock and Liquid Assets

The first Baby M trial launched a *spermatic market* in which a man's "liquid assets" wield control. The sperm provider has both money and vital fluids. The so-called surrogate has neither. She contributes mere egg and environment, the stock in this spermatic market. As stock, she is an instrument that is purchased in the manner of a transferable certificate. As stock, she is the raw material from which something, the child, is manufactured. And, as stock, she is kept for breeding purposes.

This economy, however, is not reducible simply to money and other liquid assets. It is a political economy, a *spermocracy* in which male potency is power, exercised politically against the real potency of women, whose far greater contribution and relationship to the child is rendered powerless.

In the Baby M case, the lower New Jersey court decision institutionalized new standards for measuring "real women" using the age-old stereotype of "fit mother." In doing so, it put all women on trial as mothers. It was Mary Beth Whitehead's claim to Baby Sara that was contested at the trial, not Bill Stern's. More to the point, it was Mary Beth Whitehead herself whose character was assaulted, not Bill Stern. Fortunately, the lower court decision was overturned by a higher New Jersey court, but the latter decision was limited to this one state. Unfortunately, the first Sorkow ruling has affected proposed state legislation that would make surrogate contracts legal and enforceable. Pending legislation is but one reason for examining carefully new definitions of motherhood and fatherhood that held sway in the initial decision.

Judge Sorkow based his validation of the surrogate contract, in part, on the supposed right of any woman to enter into such a transaction. But rather than a vindication of the rights of women, the court's upholding of the contract was more a punishment for any woman who would revoke her supposed natural role as mother. What invalidated Whitehead's claim to the baby was her signing of the contract. Women who sign surrogate contracts are held to a sacred and inviolable standard that no men who sign *and break* contracts every day in business and in sports, for example, have to meet. And those who deemed it scurrilous to make children the subject of a contractual exchange nevertheless insisted that Whitehead be held to the very contract they judged improper. What a pervert this woman must be, they said, who would sell her own flesh and blood for money!

Whitehead's initial "unnatural act" was reinforced by a series of more empirical "measurements." The parade of expert witnesses who were called in to gauge Whitehead's fitness for motherhood, including those who supposedly testified in her behalf, provided the damning evidence. She was accused of having a "myopic" view of motherhood and a "narcissistic personality disorder" based partly on the fact that she colored her hair. And in the most well known of such supposedly empirical standards, she was found wanting because she played patty-cake with baby Sara and gave her the wrong toys—stuffed pandas instead of pots and pans. Many experts found her fundamental flaw to be her "domination" of her husband.[3]

Judge Sorkow's decision reified this supposedly expert witness evaluation into a legal finding of fact. Sorkow found Mary Beth Whitehead to be callous and indifferent to her husband's alcohol abuse, criticizing her as "a woman without empathy." The judge also castigated her for disregarding the recommendations of her son's school district child study team, thereby "interposing herself in her son's education." He said Whitehead exploited her daughter by bringing her to the courthouse for publicity, sought to have her testify about her feelings for the baby, and thus used her children for her own "narcissistic ends" by her "fawning use of the media." As the final flaw of character, he found her to have a "genuine problem in recognizing and reporting the truth."[4] The Sorkow decision is a modern version of *The Scarlet Letter*, minus the good prose.

Sorkow's public pillaging of Mary Beth Whitehead was in stark contrast to his public praising of Bill Stern. The Sorkow decision cast Stern in the role of saint. As the son of the sole surviving members of a family who fled the Holocaust, Stern contributed to the support of his family by working at after-school jobs. His father died when Bill Stern was twelve and then, following the death of Stern's mother in 1983, "The desirability of having his own biological offspring became compelling to William Stern, thus making adoption a less desirable alternative."[5] With this short rendition of Stern's family history, a man's genetic destiny is rendered in a sympathetic light so as to make the need for biological offspring "compelling." The stage for father essentialism is not only set but furnished in a sentimental style.

The lower court ruled, "The biological father pays the surrogate for her willingness to be impregnated and carry *his* child to term. At birth, the father does not purchase the child. . . . He cannot purchase what is already his."[6] But she cannot change her mind about what is already hers because, in effect, it is his and not hers. Sperm plus money doth a father make.

The final pages of the Sorkow decision reify the ultimate ideology of father-right by chronicling what seems to be the court's finding of

Whitehead's worst failing. "To this day she still appears to reject any role Mr. Stern played in the conception. She chooses to forget that *but for him there would be no child*."[7] "But for him there would be no child." Haven't we heard this one before? These words take us back to the Aristotelian biology and ontology of man as the active principle of procreation and woman as the passive receptacle. It is he who is essential; as Simone de Beauvoir put it, woman is the essential nonessential.[8] The idea that women contribute mere matter to the child while men enspirit or ensoul the child has been a mainstay of the masculinist imagination for centuries. And the Sorkow decision illustrates that this claim for male procreative superiority is alive and well.

Father-right is also written into the language of "surrogate mother." The term privileges the male immediately. It reinforces the man as the essential, natural, biological parent while the real, natural, biological mother is rendered a mere surrogate. What's in a term? Namely, meaning. *Surrogate* means "substitute," "one who takes the place of another." A woman who gestates the fetus, experiences a nine-month pregnancy, and gives birth to the child is rendered a "substitute" mother. On the other hand, popping sperm into a jar is "real" fatherhood, legally equivalent, if not superior, to the contribution of egg, gestation, labor, and birth that is part of any woman's pregnancy.

The Sorkow decision rebiologized father-right while debiologizing mother-right. It grounded the rights of fathers in male genetic fulfillment. Male entitlement to progeny is nothing new, but, in these days of challenging the dominance of nature over nurture, we witnessed a new legal rationale for paternal natural law in the lower New Jersey court's validation of surrogate contracts. As surrogacy becomes part of the U.S. landscape, paternal essentialism translates into father-right. The father's so-called "drive to procreate"[9] prevails as a political force and "right."

The Politics of Essentialism

Many feminists who defend surrogate contracts worry that if the mother's claim to the child is recognized by law as prior and superior to the sperm source's, and if surrogate contracts are found to be legally void and unenforceable, women will be once more at the mercy of female biology. They are wary of a creeping maternal essentialism that they contend surrounds the opposition to surrogacy. What they overlook is that any defense of surrogacy will inevitably reinstitutionalize male genetic destiny, father-right, and the primacy of the spermatic market in creating a new definition of fatherhood by virtue of ejaculation. The Sorkow decision was no victory for demythologizing biology, with its recognition of the father's right to genetic fulfillment.

Yet the feminist reproductive liberal concern persists that prohibiting surrogacy will entrench motherhood in female biology and nature. For example, writer Judith Levine, in warning about the essentializing of motherhood, cautions women not to "privilege" biological sex differences by opposing surrogacy:

> Gestating a baby for nine months obviously cannot be compared to donating sperm. But does that mean, necessarily, that at birth mothers have more claim to children than fathers? Can we open up the definitions of "family"—and of men's obligations within them—without abolishing "mother-right"?[10]

Why assert male responsibility on the backs of women's rights? The language of "privileging biological sex differences" misinterprets the critical feminist claim that what is at stake in surrogacy is the creation of a breeder class of women sanctioned by the state, not a female biological essence of mothering.

Levine's opinion, like the Sorkow decision, allows a man to have a "biological bond" to a child and to create a child with a "maximum biological link" to himself. However, the same bonding is scorned, when articulated by the birthing mother, as a dangerous maternal essentialism that would take women back to the Dark Ages. The so-called surrogate must "help" in fulfilling the sperm donor's biological "drive to procreate" but is allowed no comparable claim.

Furthermore, for all the intensity of Bill Stern's "drive to procreate," he had no corresponding "drive" to rear the child. The sacrifices of daily childrearing would be assumed by the sperm provider's wife. In the aftermath of the first New Jersey court case we learned that Dr. Betsy Stern, a full-time professional pediatrician, would stay home and take care of the child. The message here is that the child will have a real and responsible mother. Dr. Stern would assume the traditional mothering location and bear the childrearing consequences of her husband's "intense drive to procreate." Surrogacy is about two women, both of whom provide mere maternal environments, doing for one man. It is a reproductive *ménage à trois,* as always with the man at the center.

There is no lack of essentialism in the surrogacy context, but feminists and others must ask where the real essentialism resides. The institution of surrogacy—and the wider proliferation of new reproductive technologies—is built upon the essentialist belief that women have a desperate need for children. More accurately, though, it seems to be men who have this essential need to perpetuate their "genetic destiny" by hiring women as surrogate breeders.

In the spermatic market of surrogate contracts, the man becomes once more the active principle of procreation, the woman is reduced to a passive conduit, and the sperm donor's wife is cast as the rejuvenated maternal principle. Together with the present social situation in which the courts increasingly privilege fathers' claims to child custody,[11] the sentimentalizing of father-child bonding in film and television, and the proliferation of fathers' rights groups, "spermocracy" prevails.

Having spent his sperm and his money, Bill Stern is entitled to what both are said to produce—the child. The ancient connotations of sperm take on particular significance in the twentieth-century context of the new reproductive technologies. Men have been preoccupied with the loss of sperm from early times, viewing their sperm as vitalistic—as a river of life—and the loss of it as a depletion of necessary energy. As the ancient ejaculator was concerned with his sperm's relation to sexuality, the modern ejaculator is additionally preoccupied with his sperm's relation to reproduction.

Motherhood as Relationship

Some opponents of surrogacy rely on maternal essentialism to argue against what they call the commodification of children. They invoke maternal instinct or maternal-infant bonding theories as a basis for outlawing surrogacy, claiming that nothing should sever the mother's biological claim to the child, especially not a contract or commercial transaction.

It is a mistake, however, to enlist motherhood essentialism in opposing surrogacy. Maternal instinct or maternal bonding arguments carry little legal weight when used in opposition to father-right. Only when motherhood essentialism is used *in the service of* father-right, as it is by the surrogate industry, does it affect court decisions and public policy.

Surrogate contracts have been interpreted as a violation of the so-called natural maternal instinct. For example, Rabbi Joseph Stern, a halachic expert in Jewish ethics and medicine and professor of Jewish law, maintains that the surrogate mother contract "contravenes the maternal instinct in womankind. . . ."[12] Richard Doerflinger, assistant director of the National Conference of Catholic Bishops Office for Pro-Life Activities, calls surrogacy "a fundamental contradiction of the maternal instinct."[13] Newspaper columnists such as A. M. Rosenthal also invoke a maternal essentialism to oppose surrogacy. A fundamental challenge to Judge Sorkow's ruling that "a deal is a deal," Rosenthal maintains, can be found in "the changes in a woman's body and mind during pregnancy that bind her to the baby. . . ."[14]

Many exsurrogates who fight bravely to retain their children, when asked why they are entitled to custody, defend their rights as mothers based on a "law of nature" or "the way God made men and women different." Mary Beth Whitehead at the founding press conference of the National Coalition Against Surrogacy stated,

> Judge Harvey Sorkow in enforcing the contract has violated nature's law. . . . Men and women are different. . . . The mother is the heart. . . . It's just the way it is.

When Patty Foster, another exsurrogate, was asked by a reporter at the same press conference what made her change her mind and revoke the surrogate contract, Foster explained, "My hormones changed."[15]

It is not surprising that this is the reasoning many women fall back on. Having been damned as unnatural mothers for giving their babies away in the first place, they rely on the rhetoric of natural motherhood to regain their children. This is the language and reasoning available to them from ages of patriarchal constructionism. It has constructed them and they in turn will reconstruct it.

It would be a mistake, however, to limit exsurrogates' opposition to surrogacy only to their words. By breaking their contracts and resisting the far greater power and resources of the ejaculatory fathers, and by their willingness to go public in the face of ridicule and lack of legal credibility, they are agents for changing women's reproductive servitude. Although they do not articulate the language of women's freedom from reproductive bondage, they embody the necessity for that freedom every time they speak out against surrogacy.

Maternal essentialism confines women to a ghetto of motherhood. Using motherhood essentialism to oppose surrogacy will not help women out of that ghetto, nor will it stop the institution of surrogacy from moving forward. Instead, it solidifies that institution by sentimentalizing the act of bearing babies for supposedly infertile persons as the greatest gift a woman could give. The defense of maternal bonding or of a maternal instinct assumes that motherhood is reducible to biology, but it is not.

Although a biological capacity, motherhood is primarily a *relationship* that occurs within a social, political, and historical context, a context that usually requires that women give of and give up themselves. Motherhood is not an instinct, a woman's essence, or a mystical state of being. Nor is it historically unchanging. Motherhood is what a given culture makes of it, and most cultures have required that women subordinate all else to this role.

Motherhood is fundamentally relational. Any woman who becomes pregnant enters into a personal and social relationship with a fetus that may become a child. This relationship is not always a positive one. Women who are forced into pregnancy against their will are not portrayed as exemplars of the maternal instinct. This is the point. Pregnancy is a relationship formed within different personal and social contexts. The relationship *may* foster significant ties between those involved, but it may not, depending on the situation. This is not to deny the intense, if often ambivalent, ties and pleasures that women feel in gestating and birthing children. This so-called bonding, however, is historically and culturally constructed and politically conditioned.

Relationships are often the basis on which legal claims can be made. The birthing mother in the surrogacy context has primary claim to the child because of her *relationship*, not just her biological link, to the child. The legal claim of the birthing mother is based on her prior and established relationship to the fetus becoming a child, which no contract can abrogate. It is also based on her personal *contribution* to the child. The woman who signs a contract to bear a child for another, even if she changes her mind, has begun to expend the energy, commitment, and work of reproduction, and it is this material contribution that governs her claim to the resultant child. Obviously, this contribution is also a bodily one. As Somer Brodribb has pointed out, we must not fear "that any reference to the female body, especially its reproductive aspects, means our condemnation as 'biological determinists,' 'dangerous essentialists'—veritable dinosaurs (mere egg-layers) outstripped by a postmodernism so androgynous there are no longer any identities or differences at all."[16]

While motherhood is, in part, a biological relationship, we must not reduce that relationship to biology. Relationships, especially those between men and women, have always been biologized. For example, sexuality has been rationalized, mostly for men, as a biological drive: "He needs it." "A natural woman puts out for a natural man." Men are often portrayed as biologically incapable of resisting what is labeled female seduction: "It was the woman, she made me do it." Women, on the other hand, are often depicted as having a masochistic biological need to be loved, thereby accepting abusive sexual acts as fulfilling this supposed essential need: "No means yes." "Every woman wants to be taken." "She asked for it."

The biologizing of sexual relationships reduces physical capabilities, feelings, and experiences, such as orgasms and breast-feeding, to instincts or drives. Physical elements and biological capacities, such as the mother's ability to feel the fetus moving in the womb, become statements about maternal instincts and bonds. It has taken centuries to begin the debiologizing of sexuality. It is time that we debiologized motherhood as well, not by technologizing or making it into a contractual issue, not by denying its location in female bodies, but by refusing its identification as female nature.

The Essentializing of the Altruistic Woman

Altruism has become part of the vocabulary of reproductive technologies and contracts. We hear about altruistic surrogacy; for example, a sister becomes pregnant for another sister with no money involved.

A mother becomes pregnant for a daughter "out of love." We even hear that women who are paid "surrogates" conceive, not mainly for the money, but primarily to give help to an infertile couple. We hear about egg donation. A woman undergoing a hysterectomy reasons that since she has no future use for her eggs, she may as well donate them to an in vitro fertilization program where they will aid an infertile woman. We hear about fetal tissue. A woman becomes pregnant with the intent of aborting for a family member who has Parkinson's disease and needs such tissue. We also hear about medically mandated, court-ordered, and postmortem cesarian sections, which are often rationalized as giving women a chance to express their altruism even in death—or just prior to it, knowing that to give birth may cause them to die.

Altruism is so accepted as a positive personal value that few question the way it has been used to legitimate many new reproductive technologies. We do not hear about the family pressure exerted on some women to become pregnant for a sister or cousin unless, like other surrogacy cases, the situation lands in court. We do not hear about the surrogate brokers who go to great lengths to soften *their* entrepreneurial image by portraying their hired "surrogates" as "special ladies" who really become pregnant for the joy of giving life to others. We do not hear about the numbers of egg donations used for embryo experimentation and genetic engineering and to further the research ambitions of reproductive scientists and technologists. We do not hear about the international traffic in fetal tissue or about the ways in which the procurement of fetal tissue for medical research adds a burden on women already facing a difficult abortion decision. And we hear little about court-ordered cesarians where the underlying norm is that the woman owes the fetus life. We do not hear about how women's altruism has become obligatory.

New reproductive technologies and arrangements are constantly portrayed in a personal context—as hope for the infertile or as resolving acute medical conditions such as Parkinson's disease or Huntington's chorea. Moreover, the discourse of altruism is appropriated by reproductive scientists to shield their objectives, interests, and ambitions; instead, the alleged miraculous technology is portrayed as bestowing a gift only dreamed of—a child, a cure, a self. Supposedly, selfless scientists engender a selfless science and technology, all for the benefit of individuals in desperate need of medical help. The alibi of altruism makes the technology beneficent, and lots more becomes acceptable.

Gifts and Gift Giving

Emphasis on women's selfless gift giving masks the complex social and political construction of women's altruism. It is always women who are called upon to be reproductive gift givers.

In his well-known study, *The Gift Relationship: From Human Blood to Social Policy*, Richard Titmuss contrasted commercial systems of maintaining a blood supply with noncommercial, altruistic systems. Titmuss's concern was to shore up the spirit of altruism and voluntarism, which he saw was declining in Western societies. In his analysis he assessed positively the possibilities of blood donation. But Titmuss also understood that giving was influenced by "the relationships set up, social and economic, between the system and the donor" and that these relationships are "strongly determined by the values and cultural orientations permeating the *donor system* and the society in general."[17] In the case of most new reproductive practices, "the donor system" mainly depends on women to donate the use of their bodies and the fruit of their wombs. It is primarily women who constitute the altruistic population called upon to contribute eggs, fetal tissue, and gestating capacities.[18]

The unexamined acceptance of women both as reproductive gifts and gift givers is deeply connected to a long-standing patriarchal tradition of giving women away in other cultural contexts—for sex and in marriage, for example. Women and women's bodies have been used as a medium of exchange and dignified as a gift throughout history. A graphic depiction of such a so-called gift occurs in the biblical text of Judges, where an old man who takes a traveler into his house is threatened by the town reprobates. Battering on the door of the man's house, they demand that the traveler, a Levite, be given over to them.

> "Send out the man who has come into your house, so that we can abuse him." Then the master of the house went out to them and said, "No, my brothers; I implore you, do not commit this crime. This man has become my guest; do not commit such an infamy. Here is my

daughter; she is a virgin; I will give her to you. Possess her, do what you please with her, but do not commit such an infamy against this man." The men would not listen to him. So the Levite took his concubine and brought her out to them. They had intercourse with her and outraged her all night till morning; when dawn was breaking they let her go. . . . In the morning . . . he saw the woman who had been his concubine lying at the door of the house. . . . He laid her across his donkey and began the journey home. Having reached his house, he picked up his knife, took hold of his concubine, and limb by limb cut her into twelve pieces; then he sent her all through the land of Israel. (Judges 19:22–30, JB)

The host protects the male guest, yet offers his daughter to appease the intruders. When they refuse the "gift" of the host's daughter, the guest offers his concubine and, after a night of sexual abuse ultimately ending in her death, carves up her body and sends it throughout the land of Israel.

This ancient story relates one tradition of gift morality that literally spreads women's bodies throughout the land, in pieces, for free. In our culture, women's personal and social obligation to give is less blatant, but it is pervasive. Women consistently give and are given to others— mostly men. This unquestioned assumption of women as givers and as given shapes the reality of reproductive gifts and gift giving. In these discussions of altruism we must continually ask: who gives and why?[19] But further, who has been given away historically and why? This is not to claim that voluntary and genuine magnanimity does not exist among women. It is to say that more is at stake than the womb, the egg, or the child as gift—and the woman as gift giver.

Technologies of Altruism?

In its appellate judgment, *In the Matter of Baby M*, the New Jersey Supreme Court found surrogate contracts contrary to the law and public policy of the state. Nonetheless, it concluded that there were no legal impediments to arrangements "when the surrogate mother volunteers, without any payment, to act as a surrogate."[20] Many state legislative committees have taken action to prohibit commercial surrogacy but are leaving untouched the whole area of noncommercial surrogate practices.

Voluntarism and altruism emerge as moral virtues in opposition to commercialism, valiantly objectifying women in their motherhood roles. Legal scholar George Annas, who has opposed commercial surrogacy, is sympathetic to the view that "one can distinguish between doing something out of love and doing it for money. As long as existing adoption laws are followed, voluntary relinquishment of a child to a close relative (such as an infertile sister) seems acceptable."[21] Such a scenario has already been played out in the setting Annas suggests.

In this country, one of the earliest publicized cases of altruistic surrogacy occurred in 1985 when Sherry King offered to become pregnant for her sister, Carole, who had undergone a hysterectomy eighteen years before. Sherry King provided both egg and womb. "I know I couldn't be a surrogate mother for money. . . . I'm doing this for love and for my sister."[22] In 1987, two Australian sisters entered an IVF surrogate arrangement (or, as it is commonly called in the United States, surrogate gestation), in which one sister, Linda Kirkman, offered to "baby-sit" (for nine months) the fertilized egg provided by her sister, Maggie Kirkman. Again, the gestating sister affirmed that it was "an act of love," and the organizing obstetrician, John Leeton, added, "The driving force was altruism, therefore I see it as a very moral and loving act."[23] Australian newspaper headlines depicted this IVF surrogate arrangement as "A Special Gift."[24]

Such altruistic surrogate agreements, however, have not been confined to sisters. In 1987, a forty-eight-year-old woman, Pat Anthony, acted as surrogate mother for her daughter, Karen, and gave birth to triplets in South Africa. Eggs were extracted from the daughter, which were fertilized in vitro with the sperm of Karen's husband, and then implanted into Karen's mother's uterus. Again, the organizing obstetrician, Dr. Bernstein, reiterated, "We feel that what Pat Anthony has done for Karen is the acceptable face of surrogacy. . . . There was no payment, no commercialism. It was an act of pure love."[25] More recently in this country, another mother, Arlette Schweitzer of Aberdeen, South Dakota, carried and birthed twins for her daughter from eggs fertilized in a laboratory dish with sperm from her daughter's husband. Described again by the media as a "labor of love," altruism was the ethical standard for an affirmative assessment of noncommercial surrogacy.[26]

Altruism also is invoked to mitigate the pecuniary perception of commercial surrogacy. Noel Keane, the well-known surrogate broker, has made an educational video called *A Special Lady*. This promotional film, which has been shown to teenage girls in high schools and other contexts, encourages them to consider "careers" as surrogates. The video cultivates the idea that it takes a special kind of woman to bear babies for others and that women who engage in surrogacy do so not mainly for the money but for the special joy it brings to the lives of those who cannot have "their own" children. The film aims to pimp young women into surrogacy using the appeal of altruism as a seasoning process—a gentle strategy of procurement casting surrogacy as a supreme act of female giving.

A 1986 article in *The Australian* used the same appeal to being special to argue "why rent-a-uterus is a noble calling." Sonia Humphrey, the author, stated,

> It does take a special kind of woman to conceive, carry under her heart and bear a child which she knows she won't see grow and develop. It also takes a special kind of woman to take a baby which is not hers by blood and rear it with all the commitment of a biological mother without the hormonal hit which nature so kindly provides. . . . But those special women do exist, both kinds. Why shouldn't both be honored?[27]

In the aftermath of the first Baby M trial in 1987, a guest editorial in the *Boston Globe* waxed euphoric. The authors, who coincidentally were "the proud parents of a beautiful daughter born to us by a surrogate mother," glorified women who "offer to bear a child for an infertile couple out of a noble combination of love and the satisfaction of knowing the joy it will bring to a new family."[28] However, as Louise Vandelac has written, "To claim that these contract-babies have been conceived through generosity, altruism, self-denial, through the love of others, or even through 'angelicism' is the only possible discourse in the early stages. Once the alibi of generosity has made the idea palatable, the rest follows, including payment, which can easily be justified as compensation or a 'return gift.'"[29]

"No woman would do this only for the money" is the cry of the surrogate brokers. The other side of this coin is that few women would do it without the money. If women were truly lining up to become surrogate mothers out of altruism and concern for the infertile, we would have middle- and upper-class women bearing the babies of lower-class couples, where the added gift of aiding those who cannot afford to pay would be an even greater expression of altruism. Presumably, altruism is a cross-class phenomenon, but it does not appear to work that way in surrogacy situations.

Researchers and clinicians go to great lengths to portray other reproductive technologies, such as "egg donations," as altruistic, too. Here, women undergoing hysterectomies or laparoscopies are urged to submit to superovulation so that multiple eggs may be extracted from them before surgery, supposedly to be used for others in later IVF procedures. As one woman—a thirty-three-year-old mother of two, from whom five eggs were taken—said, "You're having your tubes tied anyway and you don't want any more children, so even though it's some trouble, the benefits are worth it for somebody else." Journalists report that women are willing to donate "despite . . . risks and the physical and psychological screening, blood tests, sonograms and, in some cases, extra surgery they must undergo."[30] Journalists do not report, nor do doctors inform women of, *all* the risks involved, such as hyperstimulation of the ovaries, which often produces cysts and/or rupture; long-term possible cancer-causing effects from the drugs used; and chromosomal abnormalities in the donated egg cells.[31]

When complications are acknowledged, they are presented as minimal or rare, since the reality of the risks presumably might interfere with women's "altruistic" decisions.

Some women have also been asked to give fetal tissue after elective abortions for use in the experimental treatment of diseases such as Parkinson's or Huntington's chorea. Recent pleas for fetal tissue focus on its use for humanitarian medical research. The woman whose tissue is used is portrayed as helping conquer debilitating diseases. Medical research with fetal tissue has been going on for years, especially in defense-related medical experimentation, but the emphasis on the humanitarian uses of this tissue is relatively new. Donations of fetal tissue are portrayed as voluntary and altruistic, yet researchers and clinicians strongly suggest that electively aborted fetuses are "going to waste" if they cannot be used for medical research (see chapter 5).

The most-publicized cases about fetal tissue focus on women who supposedly engineer the idea of donating their fetuses. The media portrays women as the inspirational force behind the giving of fetal tissue, and when debate does take place about the ethics of fetal tissue use it is women who are frowned upon. The anti-abortionists, the ethicists, and the media worry that women will conceive with the intent of aborting for a family member or, worse, for financial gain. They point to the story of Rae Leith, spotlighted on national television in 1988, who sought to be inseminated with her father's sperm in order to treat his Alzheimer's disease. She would have conceived with the purpose of aborting so that fetal brain tissue could be transplanted into her father's brain. It was her father who said no and was portrayed as the restraining force on his daughter.[32]

However, the agency of the medical researchers and the ways in which they manipulate the ideal of women's altruism are often invisible. Take the case of Mary Ayala, for example, who became pregnant in the hope that a resultant child would yield bone marrow cells to match and save the life of her teenage daughter dying of leukemia. When her daughter Marissa was born in April 1990, her tissue did match, and the bone marrow transplant occurred in June 1991. Ayala's pregnancy raised many ethical eyebrows, but as sociologist Barbara Katz Rothman asks,

> What about the ethics of the researchers who create these dilemmas in the first place? . . . Who thought it was a reasonable thing to investigate the possibility of people as bone marrow factories for other people? Mothers didn't invent these situations, not *as* mothers.[33]

Yet mothers and pregnant women are being held ethically and legally accountable when questions arise, as if they developed the technology and dilemmas surrounding it, and the scientists fall into the benevolent background. As Katz Rothman queries, "Why don't I see *their* ethics being dissected on the nightly news? How come the ethicists aren't pontificating about *their* morality in the newspaper reports?"[34] Perhaps because the scientists and technologists have appropriated an altruistic image?

The new reproductive technologies enhance the image of science as altruistic. In vitro fertilization is represented as offering new hope for the infertile. Surrogacy gives a couple the gift of a child. Egg donation is helping others to have children. Erwin Chargaff, a molecular biologist, forcefully disputes this altruistic image, however, in stating his opposition to technological reproduction: "If the money nexus were cut so that all that now makes up reproductive technology would have to be performed without compensation, as truly samaritan deeds, if anonymity were enforced, so that all the remarkable achievements of the new applied science would have to be published without authors' names, almost all regrettable excesses would be avoided."[35]

Women's altruism is taken for granted in the pursuit of reproductive research, the advancement of reproductive science, and, of course, the giving of life. Women's altruism is called for even in death. In cases of postmortem or propemortem (near-death) obstetrical interventions, courts have ordered women's dying or dead bodies into service, mandating cesarians for the benefit of the child-to-be-born. In settings of postmortem interventions where the woman cannot consent, or in settings of near-death interventions where the woman cannot or does not consent, or where consent is questionable, altruism becomes obligatory.

The 1987 case of Angela Carder, a twenty-eight-year-old pregnant woman dying of cancer, is illustrative. In an emergency hearing set up in the hospital as Angela Carder lay dying, the judge—over Angela Carder's final expressed objection to undergoing the surgery—ordered that her twenty-six-week-old fetus be delivered by cesarian section. The grounds for this decision seemed to rest on the principle that the life of the fetus outweighed any interest Angela Carder might have in her own life or health—*because* she was dying. The baby died two hours after she was born, and Angela Carder died two days later after having been treated as though she were already dead. Her parents contend that the cesarian hastened her death by making her physical condition worse.

The lawyer for the fetus, Barbara Mishkin, who was appointed by the court, said she was "convinced then and I'm convinced now . . . that this woman wanted that baby. She risked her life for that baby."[36] Barbara Mishkin was convinced that Angela Carder gave her life so that others might live. In the majority of these near-death or after–brain death reproductive interventions, it is increasingly the courts, the lawyers, and in some cases the doctors who express the expected altruism of the women involved.[37]

Many critics have pointed to the exceptional standards applied in this and in other cases of forced cesarians where pregnant women are treated against their will. Pregnant women function as the only patients who cannot refuse extraordinary treatment to save others. Outside the context of procreation and pregnancy, sick or dying patients cannot be forced to give organs or bone marrow or even blood for a person whose life can only be saved by their particular donations. Why then are pregnant women the exception to the rule? As philosopher Caroline Whitbeck has stated in a different context, "The moral expectation upon women is that they be nurturant, that is, that they ought to go beyond respecting rights and meet the needs of others. . . ."[38] In the case of pregnant women, the moral expectation that women meet the needs of others is greater to the extent that the woman is expected to sacrifice her own health and life for that of the fetus.

The expectation of women's altruism is most evident in situations of postmortem ventilation (PMV), where the pregnant woman's vital functions are maintained by artificial means in order to allow the fetus to grow and develop to a presumed sustainable age. Some women's bodies have been kept in a ventilated state for several months to bring the fetus to term. In one 1986 case, a brain-dead woman was kept alive for seven weeks so that her twenty-one-week-old fetus would have a chance to survive. This was done at the request of a man who claimed to be the father of the fetus, against the wishes of the woman's husband. The court accepted the argument that the woman's right of privacy no longer applied since she was dead and the state now had a dominant interest in protecting human life.[39] Three months premature, the baby died shortly after a cesarian delivery was performed, when the fetal heartbeat suddenly weakened; the woman's body, removed from life support systems, died shortly thereafter. As philosopher Julien Murphy has commented, "The practice of PMV suggests that its proponents do not believe that maternal brain activity is a requirement for pregnancy. . . . To imagine a dead woman's body as 'artificially' pregnant is to claim that women in pregnancy are essentially 'pregnant bodies'. . . that a woman's connection to her pregnancy is neither vital nor necessary." Murphy points out that the woman's body thus becomes a "natural" life support machine for the fetus, denying brain-dead women the right to an immediate bodily death.[40] When PMV is imposed on brain-dead pregnant women, the expectation is that women must give life even in death, the supreme act of female giving historically being maternal death in childbirth. As women and women's bodies are expected to be support systems in life, so too in death.

If postmortem ventilation is permitted, why not postmortem ventilation surrogacy? In other words, brain-dead women, their bodies kept alive by artificial means, could be used as incubators for someone else's embryos in the same way that brain-dead women are kept alive to grow their own fetuses to term and as bodies are now ventilated for organ donations and transplants. This is exactly what was proposed in 1988 by an Australian bioethicist, Paul Gerber, from Queensland University. Dr. Gerber said, "The idea to use the brain dead and neomorts—newly dead people—was not ghoulish and was better than commercial surrogacy" because "at least the dead would be doing some good." After these dead women have been used as surrogates they could be used for organ transplants. "It's a wonderful solution for the problems posed by surrogacy, and a magnificent use of a corpse."[41]

The proposal, reported to have been discussed seriously at medical conferences in Australia, generated debate and disgust from many, including the Victorian premier, John Cain, on the grounds that it was abhorrent to turn dead bodies into objects for the use of others. Yet Mr. Cain, who was willing to change Australia's adoption law to accommodate the IVF surrogacy case between the two Kirkland sisters in Victoria,[42] obviously thought it proper that live female bodies be turned into objects for the use of others as long as such bodies are given freely out of love.

Altruism holds sway. Part of its dominance as an ethical norm derives from its opposition to commercialism. Particularly in the United States, opponents of legalizing surrogate contracts contend that these contracts make children into commodities to be bought and sold. Many have also focused on the *economic exploitation* of the women in financial need who enter surrogate contracts. In these perspectives, the ethical objection is restricted to the fact that a price tag is attached to that which should have no price. The alternative, they argue, is surrogacy for free, which is morally and legally appropriate, especially when it is kept within the family. Without money involved, the reproductive altruism of women is not only morally appropriate, but morally celebrated.

The Moral Celebration of Women's Altruism

The cultural norm of the altruistic woman who is infinitely giving and eternally accessible derives from a social context in which women give and are given away, but also from a moral tradition that celebrates women's duty to meet and satisfy the needs of others. The cultural expectation of altruism has fallen most heavily on pregnant women; they are the archetypal altruists. Ethicist Beverly Wildung Harrison notes the essentialism of this assumption about women's altruism: "Many philosophers and theologians, although decrying gender inequality, still unconsciously assume that women's lives should express a different moral norm than men's, that women should exemplify moral purity and self-sacrifice, whereas men may live by the more minimal rational standards of moral obligation. . . . Perfection and self-sacrifice are never taken to be a day-to-day moral requirement for any moral agent except, it would seem, a pregnant woman."[43]

Harrison calls this a "superogatory morality," acts that are expected to go beyond the accepted standards of obligation. While traditionally women are exhorted to be passive, simultaneously women are expected to be more responsible than men for meeting the needs of others: "We live in a world where many, perhaps most, of the voluntary sacrifices on behalf of human well-being are made by women, but the assumption of a special obligation to self-giving or sacrifice . . . is male-generated ideology."[44]

The other side of the altruistic coin is male self-interest. A man is allowed to be self-seeking, to go to great lengths to fulfill his self-interests; we have seen this self-interest rationalized, in the case of surrogacy, as genetic continuity and biological fulfillment. Philosopher Sarah Hoagland goes further and makes the point that the more dominant a man's self-seeking, the greater a role woman's altruism must play. Women's "altruism and self-sacrifice is reinforced and heightened by the excesses of men and the state, and we turn to the idea of women as essentially altruistic and self-sacrificial (nurturing, unconditionally loving, and so on) in a romantic desperation for assurance of the possibility of grace and goodness in this world."[45] This is not an ideological pronouncement about female self-giving and male self-seeking, but an essentialism that defines the reality of daily life imposed on many women. As such, it raises complex questions about moral double standards in a cultural context where men as a class set the standards and women live them out; where inequality is systemic; and where women have an investment in their own subordination. This does not mean that every man is self-interested and every woman altruistic. Were that the case, surely the biological determinists would be right!

Moreover, a distinct moral language accompanies the tradition that celebrates women's essential altruism. It is the language of selflessness and responsibility toward others in which women's very possibilities are framed. It is the discourse of maternalism, which traditionally has equated devotion and dedication with women abandoning their own needs. It is also the discourse of maternal destiny in which a real woman is a mother or one who acts like a mother or, more specifically, one who acts like the self-sacrificing, nurturant, and caretaking mother a woman is supposed to be. And with altruistic surrogacy, it is the discourse of providing families and children for others. If a woman chooses a different destiny and directs her self elsewhere, she risks placing herself outside female nature *and* culture.

A body of recent feminist literature, most notably the work of psychologist Carol Gilligan, has valorized women's altruistic development as the morality of responsibility, emphasizing that this is morality "in a different voice" from that of men.[46] Formerly a mainstay of separate but equal ideology, as in "vive la différence," this same discourse is now being transformed by some feminists into an endorsement of women's difference in human and moral development. Yet, as legal theorist Catharine MacKinnon notes,

> For women to affirm difference, when difference means dominance, as it does with gender, means to affirm the qualities and characteristics of powerlessness. . . . So I am critical of affirming what we have been, which necessarily is what we have been permitted. . . . Women value care because men have valued us according to the care we give them. . . .[47]

Altruism has been one of the most effective blocks to women's self-awareness and demand for self-determination, serving, like mothering, as an essential instrument that structures social organization and patterns of relationship in women's lives. The discourse of altruism has also

legitimated women's servile self-sacrifice. The social relations organized around norms of altruism and the giving of self are powerful
forces that bind women to patriarchal roles and expectations. When
exercised from a subordinate position in the interests of a super-
ordinate class, however, altruism is not a virtue. Furthermore, the very
virtue of altruism grows out of the context of women's subordination.
As philosopher Mary Daly long ago pointed out, "Part of the problem
with this moral ideology is that it became accepted not by men but by
women, who hardly have been helped by an ethic which reinforces the
abject female situation."[48]

The issue is not whether altruism can have any positive place in the
lives of women, but rather that we cannot abstract this question from
the gender-specific and unequal situation of women and the patriarchal
values and structures in which new reproductive practices are arranged. Altruism is not crudely obligatory. The issue is what kind of
choices women can make within the context of a patriarchal culture and
tradition that orients them to give and give of themselves.

Nonetheless, when feminists stress how women's choices are limited by the social system and how women are channeled into giving,
feminists are reproached for portraying women as passive victims. Lori
Andrews in her essay, "Alternative Modes of Reproduction," for the
Reproductive Laws for the 1990s handbook, faults feminist critics of the
new reproductive technologies for embracing arguments based on "a
presumed incapacity of women to make decisions."[49] For Andrews,
pressure seems to exist only at the barrel of a gun. This reductionistic
view has been challenged by many, including the New Jersey Supreme
Court, which reversed the trial court's decision in the Whitehead-Stern
surrogacy case. To its credit, the court recognized the complexity of
consent in its assessment that for the so-called surrogate, money is an
"inducement" as is the "coercion of contract." Many so-called feminists
refuse to acknowledge the same inducements, preferring to represent
women as unproblematically choosing their fate in highly problema-
tized contexts (see chapter 3).

For women, gift giving is a source of identity, status, and relief from
guilt. Women who don't give—time, energy, care, sex—are exposed to
disapproval or penalty. But the more important element here is that on
a cultural level women *are expected* to donate themselves in the form
of time, energy, and body, particularly as mothers.

Sociologist Emile Durkheim, in his classic work on suicide, maintained that suicide, seemingly the most individual of acts, must be viewed as the result of certain facts of the social milieu, what he called *courants suicidogènes.* One of these social currents was altruism. Durkheim discussed altruistic suicide as the manifestation of a *conscience collective,* the capacity of group values and forces to supersede the claims of individuality and, in the case of soldiers and widows, for example, to influence a tendency to suicide. Durkheim observed that altruistic suicide involved a group attachment of great strength, such that individual assertion and fulfillment and even life itself became secondary. The ego was given over to and eventually absorbed in another, having been stripped of its individuality. Altruism resulted when social integration was strong, so binding that the individual became not only absorbed in the group but in the group's expectations.[50]

Durkheim's analysis of social integration is especially applicable to the social construction of women's altruism. For women, family expectations often generate a powerful force for social integration, with family values and inducements overriding a woman's individuality. This is especially evident in the context of family surrogacy arrangements.

Family Ties, Gifts, and the Inducement of Altruism

The use of multiple women in families for reproduction is grounded in many religious patriarchal traditions. Men took an array of wives and concubines, not only for sex but also to reproduce. The reproductive use of multiple women was culturally and religiously legitimated as extended family, otherwise known as polygyny. In ancient Israel, for example, a large family, in particular a large number of sons, was regarded as a blessing from Yahweh. The desire for progeny was partially responsible for the system of multiple wives and concubinage. Surrogacy, especially family surrogacy, replicates this model, with the man inseminating a female family member in order to reproduce "his issue." As one commentator noted, we are really talking not only about surrogate mothers, but about "surrogate wives."[51]

The potential for women's exploitation is not necessarily less when no money is involved and reproductive arrangements take place among family members. In fact, the family is the least safe place for women. More women are sexually abused, battered, and killed in the family context than anyplace else. Yet most of the literature on family surrogacy—sisters bearing children for sisters, for example—romanticizes the family as the foremost place of protection. However, unique affective "inducements" exist in familial contexts that do not exist elsewhere. Although there is no legal "coercion of contract" or perhaps no "inducement" of money, there could be the coercion of family ties, in which having a baby for a sister or another family member may be rationalized as the "greatest gift" one woman can give to another. In these family situations, sisterhood becomes surrogacy; that is, sister love is equated with one sister becoming pregnant for her sibling. Yet, rather than surrogacy enhancing sisterhood, is it not exploiting a sister to put her at risk physically and psychologically? As one woman wrote, "What kind of a society do we live in, that would condone women using other women in this way?"[52]

Gifts often have an operative role and power in shaping family life, as in social life in general. In *The Gift: Forms and Functions of Exchange in Archaic Societies*, anthropologist Marcel Mauss contends that gifts fulfill certain obligations. These obligations vary, but in all instances, whether gifts are used to maintain social affection or to promote unity or loyalty within the group, they are experienced in some way as prescriptive and exacting.[53] This is true on a cultural level, as Mauss has pointed out, but it is even more true on a family level, the context most often cited as the desirable site of altruistic reproductive exchanges.

Family opinion may not force a woman, in the sense of being outrightly coercive, to become pregnant for another family member. Where family integration is strong, however, the nature of family opinion may be so engulfing that, for all practical purposes, it exacts a reproductive donation from a female source. When a surrogate arrangement is represented as generosity to a family member in need, the ideal of altruism binds the woman to the norms of family duty.

Within families, it may be considered selfish, uncaring, and even dishonorable for a woman to deprive a relative of eggs, fetal tissue, or her gestating abilities. The category of altruism itself is *broadened* in family contexts to include all sorts of nontraditional reproductive duties that would be frowned on if women did these for money. Within families, it may be considered selfish for an infertile woman to deprive her husband of children by not allowing the use of another female family member, especially *because* the arrangements will be kept within the family.

It is also likely that those with less power in the family will be expected to be more altruistic. Indeed, their altruism may be outrightly coerced, as happened to Alejandra Muñoz. Muñoz, a poor, illiterate Mexican woman, was brought across the U.S. border illegally to bear a child for relatives at the urging of family members. Told by relatives that if she became pregnant the embryo would be flushed out and transferred to the womb of her cousin, Muñoz was deceived about her reproductive role. When this embryo transfer did not happen, Muñoz vowed to end the pregnancy and was thwarted by family members who kept her under house confinement until the delivery. When she fought to keep her child, she was threatened with exposure as an illegal alien.[54]

In family surrogate arrangements, relatives do the brokering. Family members are inevitably used as essential intermediaries and gatekeepers between the woman and the would-be recipients of a child. And women are still negotiated by family agents, whether for money or for free. We should also not assume that, because surrogate arrangements occur within the family context, no money changes hands. Increasingly many relatives accept a "return gift" for their services. In the realm of organ donations, by comparison, Dr. James Light of the Washington (D.C.) Hospital Center, one of the nation's largest transplant centers, estimates that some economic benefit accrues to 15 to 20 percent of living organ donors who give to a relative.[55]

Altruism, Law, and Public Policy

In 1989 a New Jersey State Task Force on New Reproductive Practices recommended that unpaid surrogate arrangements between friends, relatives, or others be made legally unenforceable. One task force member directed her criticism of noncommercial surrogacy to the family context. Arguing that surrogate arrangements between family members portend the same "disastrous implications" as the Baby M contract, Emily Arnow Alman said that she could foresee the "not-so-bright cousin being exploited to bear a child for a relative."[56]

We might ask further what is suitable matter for exchange. When the media speak of reproductive gifts and donations, especially where the gift and donation is the woman's body and the child who may be born of such a practice, the donation of persons is put on a par with the exchange of objects. The woman and child become gift-objects. The director of the New Jersey Task Force stated, "The task force feels that the state shouldn't confer any imprimatur of legitimacy on the practice of surrogacy in any form" and that "treating women and children and limiting their liberty by contracts enforceable by the state makes them less than human beings."[57]

The only country thus far to have invalidated all forms of surrogacy is Australia. The ministers of health and social welfare from all the Australian states united to adopt a uniform approach to surrogacy legislation, concluding that surrogacy involved "a risk of harm to parties and that there are substantial uncertainties attached to the practice as a means of family formation."[58] Recognizing that a consistent and uniform approach to surrogacy was needed, the ministers agreed that "there were too many unknowns, too many uncertainties and that we oughtn't experiment with the creation of children. . . . People who go this way . . . should not be supported by the community."[59] They rejected the views of the National Bioethics Consultative Committee that these unknowns and uncertainties would be minimized by regulation and found "that any system for regulation of surrogacy inherently serves to promote and institutionalize the practice rather than deter it." The social welfare and health ministers specifically recognized that surrogacy leaves women and children open to exploitation.[60] Although Australia has been in the forefront of new reproductive experimentation on women, this legislation shows the power of feminist advocacy, particularly the work of Australian FINRRAGE, against new reproductive expansionism.

Reproductive gift relationships must be seen in a political as well as a familial context. Egg donation, the giving of fetal tissue, and noncommercial surrogacy cannot be treated as pure acts of altruism; moral meaning and public policy should not be governed by the mere absence of market values. But moral meaning and public policy should be guided by the specificity of gender. What does this mean? For one thing, it means that any ethical or legal assessment of reproductive gifts *begins*

with the realization that women are both gift and gift giver. The validation of altruistic surrogacy, on the level of public policy, leaves intact
the image and reality of a woman as a *reproductive conduit*, someone
through whom someone passes. State legislative committees, with the
exception of the New Jersey task force, have generally approved of
altruistic noncommercial surrogacy arrangements, thereby affirming
the norm of women's altruism in the reproductive context. A gender-
specific lens challenges this generalist affirmation of women's reproductive altruism and makes explicit the consequences for women.

Whether a woman serves as an egg, fetal tissue, or maternal vehicle,
she is demeaned as a person and becomes a generous tool, renamed a
reproductive gift. Whether money is involved or not, she is still an
instrument of exchange. Thus the terminology of *donor* is inaccurate,
and women are more appropriately *sources* of eggs, fetal tissue, and
babies, and we are not really talking about *donations* but about *procurement*, albeit friendly and familial.

Surrogacy, situated within the larger context of women's inequality,
is not simply about the commercialization of women and children. On
a political level, it reinforces the perception and use of women as a
breeder class and the gender inequality of women as a group. The practice of surrogacy strikes at the core of what a society allows women to
be and become. Taking the commerce out of surrogacy but leaving the
practice intact on a noncommercial and contractual basis glosses over
the essential violation—the social definition of women as breeders. This
is not symbolic or intangible, because the image of woman as reproductive object, like the image of woman as sexual object, is entrenched in
most societies. As women's studies student Carol Mc Master wrote,
"Forced reproduction has been a continuum on a grand scale throughout history, usually with no money involved. . . . Commercial surrogacy
is highly industrialized reproductive exploitation; altruistic surrogacy,
highly personalized exploitation."[61]

Proposals that the law keep clear of reproductive exchanges where
no money changes hands are based on unreal gender-neutral assumptions. If the harm of surrogacy, for example, is based only on the commercialization and commodification of reproduction, then the reality
that *women* are always used in systems of surrogacy gets no legal notice.
While it may seem an obvious fact that no one other than women can

be exploited as surrogates, this so-called fact is not recognized in legislation. As a matter of public policy, the violation of a woman's person, dignity, and integrity have received no legal standing in most legislation
opposed to surrogacy other than as mere allusion (the New Jersey Task
Force recommendations are a notable exception). By not giving the violation of women primary standing in legislation opposing commercial
surrogacy, women's systematic inequality is made invisible and kept in
place. That inequality can then be dignified as noble in so-called altruistic arrangements.

The focus on altruism essentializes the woman as gift giver and
as gift. It sentimentalizes and thus obscures the ways women are medicalized and devalued by the new reproductive technologies and practices. An uncritical affirmation of reproductive gifts and gift givers—
of egg donation, of "special ladies" who serve as so-called surrogate
mothers for others, and of reproductive technology itself as a great
gift to humanity—fails to examine the institutions of reproductive science, technology, and brokering that increasingly structure reproductive exchanges.

Altruistic reproductive exchanges leave intact the status of women
as a breeder class, whether for producing eggs, fetal tissue, or babies.
Women's bodies are still the raw material for others' needs, desires, and
purposes. The normalization of altruistic exchanges may, in fact, have
the effect of further promoting the view that women have a duty or
obligation to engage in reproductive arrangements free of charge. In the
surrogacy context, altruism essentializes the role of women as *mothers
for others*. This emphasis on giving has become an integral part of
reproductive technological propaganda, but this altruistic pedestal on
which women are placed is only one more way of glorifying women's
inequality.

Equal Rights?

Inequality takes many forms, but one of its most deceptive faces shows
pseudosymmetries between women and men. False equivalents, often
proclaimed as equal rights, abound in discussions of reproductive technologies. One of the most superficial notions that has surfaced in the
surrogacy debate is that sperm is equal to egg, gestation, and birthing.

In the Sorkow decision, the "equalizers" went so far as to declare that the male genetic contribution superseded the female genetic, gestational, and generative contributions. But the male relationship and contribution to the fetus-becoming-a-child are not equal to the female's. The sperm provider does not assume the risks of conception, pregnancy, and birth, nor does he do the work of carrying the fetus for nine months. His is a spermatic contribution—one of genes alone, prior to any parenting relationship. To ignore a birthing mother's more substantive relational claim and to disregard her far greater material contribution to the fetus is to reduce her to a mechanized object, thus creating a new traffic in women as commodities to be bought and sold for breeding purposes.

We see this same equalizing practice at work in disputes over frozen embryos. In 1989, in a U.S. State Circuit Court in Knoxville, Tennessee, a divorced couple fought over embryos that had been frozen in a warmer time. The man, Junior Davis, wanted the embryos disposed of, and the woman, Mary Sue Davis, wanted the embryos thawed and implanted in her body.

Some experts argued that both parents had equal rights to the embryos. In contrast, Mary Sue Davis argued that her legal claim to the embryos was based on the rights of the embryos as "preborn children" to life. She did not argue for any rights of her own based, for example, on her greater contribution to the embryos, a contribution that had entailed a considerable personal investment of repeated and painful attempts at implantation and gestation.

Junior Davis was not so modest about asserting his equal rights. He maintained that the embryos should *not* be implanted and born because this would violate his right to control his reproduction.[62] In stronger language, he even contended that he was being "raped of [his] reproductive rights."[63] In what sounded like a new male entitlement to abortion, Junior Davis argued he would be forced into fatherhood if the embryos were implanted and carried to term, even though he would not be bearing the physical, emotional, or financial responsibility.

Maintaining that his self-interest in *not* becoming a father was paramount in preventing his exwife from thawing their frozen embryos, Davis sued for veto power over the disposition of the embryos. Testifying at the trial as an expert witness, John Robertson, legal champion of "procreative liberty," avowed that the case should be decided in favor of Mr. Davis because he would be hurt more by losing. In reported testimony that displayed callous ignorance of the invasive and interventionist procedures that women must endure in order to engender frozen embryos, Robertson argued that Mrs. Davis could try another in vitro fertilization program if she lost the case, which would be "less of a burden" on her than unwanted fatherhood on Mr. Davis.[64]

A closer look at this "lesser burden" reveals that Mary Sue Davis underwent five tubal pregnancies resulting in the rupture of one fallopian tube and the tying of the other before entering the in vitro fertilization program in Knoxville, Tennessee. This is a common condition of many women who resort to in vitro fertilization. Prior to IVF, they have experienced many pregnancy failures and painful interventions, such as fertility treatments and workups, which often include blowing out their tubes with gas. Then they undergo the interventions of an in vitro fertilization program—fertility drugs, laparoscopies to extract the eggs, and, most often, failed implantations of the eggs after external fertilization in the petri dish. Mary Sue Davis had two unsuccessful implantations.

Furthermore, it should be noted that Mary Sue Davis wanted no parental support or assistance from her exhusband. She elected to raise the child, if born, on her own. To this, Junior Davis responded that he did not want a child of his—the child he did not want born but yet wants to control—reared in a single-parent household. Adding another dimension of father-right to the legal picture was that of the medical progenitor, Dr. I. Ray King, who runs the in vitro program used by Davis. King said that he would not consent to Mary Sue Davis using donated sperm for additional IVF attempts after her divorce and, further, would not allow a single woman into the program. This attitude is in keeping with the restrictions in most IVF programs limiting procedures to those who are heterosexual and married.

Increasingly, the medical "fathers," the IVF clinics, are asserting ownership rights over frozen embryos—precious commodities in the world of IVF and genetic engineering research. In another frozen embryo dispute that did not receive as much publicity as the Davis case, Risa and Steven York took the in vitro fertilization program at the Jones Institute in Norfolk, Virginia, to court. After Risa York underwent three failed implants, the couple decided to freeze the resulting embryos. The couple then moved to California and wanted their frozen embryos shipped to the Good Samaritan Hospital in Los Angeles, where Risa York would undergo another implantation under the supervision of Dr. Richard Marrs. But Dr. Howard Jones of the Norfolk clinic refused the transfer, saying that the Yorks had no rights to the embryos outside his institute's jurisdiction.

In what became a turf dispute among the various medical men involved, Richard Marrs took aim at his competitors: "When a physician starts owning embryos and making decisions for his patients, there'll be no stopping anyone who has anything to do with pregnancy from getting involved."[65] The point seems lost on Marrs that the whole history of reproductive technologies thus far has been for the physician to usurp more and more decisions about pregnancy and birth from women. This case was finally settled in the federal district court in Virginia, which held in 1989 that the Norfolk clinic held the embryos in bailment (trust) pending their use in an IVF cycle. Once the Yorks wanted to transfer their remaining embryo out of state, the clinic's bailment was finished and the Norfolk clinic was compelled to transfer the embryo to the California center.[66]

In the Davis embryo-freezing dispute, the spotlight was on the rights of sperm providers, "ejaculatory fathers," and medical "fathers." Nobody spoke about women's rights, not even Mary Sue Davis. Instead, Jay Christenberry, her lawyer, argued that embryos are preborn children. He enlisted the testimony of a French geneticist who declared that life begins at conception because that is when the human genetic blueprint is fixed. And then came the initial lower court decision. On September 21, 1989, Judge Dale Young, concluding that the frozen embryos were in fact "human beings existing as embryos," awarded custody of the seven frozen embryos to Mary Sue Davis. One is tempted to say that the right conclusion was reached for the wrong reason, but this would be too simplistic.

Mary Sue Davis won the first legal battle by arguing that the embryos were persons, an argument no doubt advised by her lawyers who sensed the fetalist[67] political climate and took advantage of it. They gambled that fetal personhood and rights stood on more secure legal ground than women's personhood and rights. Women, like Mary

Sue Davis, are catching on that an argument for fetal status and rights is more likely to succeed.

Even arguing for fetal rights, however, did not ultimately benefit Mary Sue Davis. On appeal, the embryo ruling was overturned. The Tennessee Court of Appeals supposedly "equalized" the lower court's decision by granting joint custody of the embryos to both Mary Sue Davis (remarried and now Mary Sue Davis Stowe) and Junior Davis. As the court stated, "It would be repugnant and offensive to constitutional principles to order Mary Sue to implant these fertilized ova against her will. It would be equally repugnant to order Junior to bear the psychological, if not the legal, consequences of paternity against his will."[68] Finally, in 1992 Tennessee's highest court ruled that Junior Davis could prevent his exwife from using or donating the frozen embryos since, through implantation or donation, Mr. Davis would be robbed of his procreative right to avoid parenthood. The court held that if one party does not want to become a parent, his or her interest always outweighs the other's interest in the disposition of the embryos unless the other party cannot become a parent in any way.[69] The irony of this decision is that it upholds a *man's* right not to become a parent against his will. As we have seen in forced cesarian cases and in the age-old abortion debate, the law has been quite willing to compel women to do what this court was not willing to compel a man to do.

One lesson of the Davis case is that women and women's rights are considerably diminished by new reproductive "options." Mary Sue Davis's initial victory was no victory for women, since fetal rights are almost always set in opposition to women's rights. Moreover, when the Tennessee Court of Appeals granted both parties joint custody of the embryos, Mary Sue Davis had changed her marital status and her mind, choosing now to donate the embryos anonymously to an infertile couple. Junior Davis then argued that his exwife's change of mind weakened her case and that donating the embryos was even less acceptable to him than having his exwife in control of them.

When Fetal Rights Equals "Fathers'" Rights

Fathers' rights are increasingly being asserted in the thin guise of fetal rights. Activist and writer John Stoltenberg contends that "the fetus as penis" has symbolically and materially dominated any reproductive forum. "Men control women's reproductive capacities in part because men believe that fetuses are phallic—that the ejaculated leavings swelling up in utero are a symbolic and material extension of the precious penis itself. This belief is both literal and metaphorical, both ancient and modern."[70] In litigation involving new reproductive technologies, we have seen that ejaculation confers father-right.

Ejaculatory fathers' rights are also becoming quite prominent in abortion cases, where the inseminator challenges a woman's right to proceed with an abortion. In the United States, for example, several cases have reached the courts. The boyfriend of an eighteen-year-old pregnant Indiana woman won a court order forbidding her to have an abortion. Arguing that he would pay her medical expenses and raise the child-to-be, he thus claimed that his rights outweighed hers. Before the court could rule on this case, the woman had an abortion, but the court did find in favor of the male petitioner stating, "The rights of the father in his unborn children are of constitutional dimensions under the 14th and 9th Amendments to the U.S. Constitution as well as being derived from the Indiana common law. Those constitutional rights of the father outweigh the constitutional rights of the mother."[71] In New York, a man sued for divorce and money because his wife had an abortion without his consent. He asserted that this was a case of "fathers' rights." He also sued the doctors and hospital where the abortion was performed.[72]

One of the most publicized abortion cases ensued when Canada's Supreme Court went into emergency session in August 1989 to decide whether a Quebec woman, Chantal Daigle, could be restrained by her former abusive boyfriend, Jean-Guy Tremblay, from having an abortion. In this case, Jean-Guy Tremblay argued that his self-interest in becoming a father was paramount in preventing his former girlfriend from having an abortion and thereby protecting the fetus. In their relationship he had gone to great lengths to ensure his paternity, even ordering her to stop using contraceptives when they tentatively planned marriage. Tremblay himself was reported to have testified that he substituted other tablets for Daigle's birth control pills when she refused to stop using them.[73]

Tremblay's "self-interest" in becoming a father, however, was transformed into the state's interest in defending the fetus. Jean-Guy Tremblay's lawyer, Robert Francis, showed an anti-abortion film to the

Canadian Supreme Court intended to portray the fetus as a human being with all the rights of a person. Referring to the 1989 U.S. *Webster v. Reproductive Services* ruling, which gave states the right to limit and regulate abortions within their own jurisdictions, Francis said, "The Supreme Court decision of the United States gave us all the hope."[74] Meanwhile, Jean-Guy Tremblay had written a will, leaving his property to the fetus. Jean-Guy maintained that stealing his lover's contraception was okay; abusing her while she was pregnant was okay; but abortion is not okay because the fetus has the right to the protection of paternity.

As fetal rights begin to dominate the reproductive agenda of this country, we must examine the ways in which ejaculatory fathers' rights are articulated under the heading of fetal rights, and women's rights are diminished under this same banner. Fortunately, the Supreme Court of Canada struck down the lower court's injunction prohibiting Daigle from having an abortion, ruling unanimously that the injunction could not be upheld. Prior to the Supreme Court's decision, however, Daigle's lawyer announced that she had proceeded with the abortion despite the injunction. It is disturbing to note that in this case the injunction issued to prevent Daigle from having an abortion was upheld by two lower courts before it reached Canada's Supreme Court. At that time, she was twenty-three weeks pregnant. It is reported that there are also at least three other men who have obtained injunctions in provincial courts to stop their lovers from having abortions.[75]

One of the strategies of groups seeking to outlaw abortion in Canada is to link rights for prospective fathers to the rights of fetuses. Anti-abortion agitators have increased demonstrations and have won places on governing boards of hospitals, and they credit the latter with preventing a number of abortions in British Columbia. Their tactics include seeking civil court rulings to establish the rights of "fathers" to protect the rights of fetuses.

The Canadian case and the 1989 U.S. Supreme Court decision on *Webster v. Reproductive Services* demonstrate that abortion and the new reproductive technologies are inextricably linked. North American women are once again confronting the issue of abortion, in part, *because the advent of and publicity given to the new reproductive technologies has created a social context and perception in which the rights of sperm providers and fetuses have become paramount.* And as the ejaculatory father emerges as the protector of the fetus, fathers' rights merge with fetal rights.

In the panoply of many new reproductive technologies—in vitro fertilization, embryo experimentation, transfer, and freezing, and fetal tissue transplantation—we see the *separability and severability* of the embryo/fetus from the woman. As the new reproductive technologies increasingly separate and sever the fetus/embryo from the woman, the medical progenitors create an adversarial relationship between woman and fetus. Even when the fetus is still in the womb, doctors often become police officers of the pregnancy, reporting alleged abusive behavior from the mother, for example, alcohol and drug intake or refusal to submit to a cesarian. They monitor any female activity that is judged harmful to the fetus, *not any medical interventions that might harm the pregnant woman.* Women are expected to submit to any directives or any invasive, painful, and unnecessary technology that doctors judge necessary to protect or improve the quality of the fetus. Since July 1989, when the U.S Supreme Court gave the states broader authority to limit abortion, ten more fetal abuse cases have been filed against women in the United States.

If the fetus becomes the primary "patient" while still in the womb, how much more so when it is detached from the woman's body in procedures where fetuses can be grown, frozen, and thawed technologically. Modern obstetrical practice has confirmed the pregnant woman as mere maternal environment for the fetus. Surrogacy has confirmed the pregnant woman as incubator for someone else's child-to-be-born. And other new reproductive techniques such as IVF and embryo transfer confirm the woman as egg producer or baby machine.

It is no surprise then that in the 1990s, fetal rights are in the foreground. This is due not only to the activism of conservative and fundamentalist right wing groups, like Operation Rescue, but also to reproductive liberals who promote the development of and access to invasive new reproductive technologies. Those who care about women's reproductive rights are fundamentally nearsighted when they focus only on the glare of the anti-abortion movement without looking beyond to the more dimly lit scene of pro-reproductive technology liberalism.

Disputes like the Davis case, in which embryos are frozen, not only situate the fetus in its own right but give centrality to the sperm provider as well. The ground is then fertilized for the growth of the reproductive rights of ejaculators under the banner of gender equality. As Charles Clifford, the lawyer for Junior Davis, phrased it, "If we are ever to make men truly equal partners, you can't just say that because she is female, she has greater rights."[76]

Reducing Motherhood to Fatherhood

As the definition and rights of fathers are expanded by new reproductive technologies and contracts, the definition and rights of mothers shrink. Consider the 1990 surrogate gestation case in which a supposedly new form of surrogacy was widely publicized—called "pure" surrogacy, as if it had been blessed by Mother Teresa. Anna Johnson, an African American, bore a child for Mark Calvert, a white man, and his wife, Christina Calvert, an Asian American. For the public, the newness of this case was that the so-called surrogate did not provide the egg and thus, as the newspapers represented it, the baby "has no biological relation to her."[77]

In this case, motherhood was reduced to the most attenuated component of female reproduction—an egg. The California court decision awarded custody of the child to the gamete providers, the Calverts, and in so doing affirmed that genetics was the primary criterion of parenthood. The lawyer for Anna Johnson argued that the woman who gives birth is the natural, biological, and legal mother. The lawyer for the Calverts, as well as the baby's court-appointed attorney, argued that genetics has been consistently used by the courts to determine parenthood and that the so-called surrogate was a mere custodian. Or, as Orange County Superior Court Judge Richard N. Parslow, Jr., opined, pregnancy is comparable to foster care.[78]

The view of the Calverts and the judge is consistent with the way that courts and legislation have continually perceived motherhood, pregnancy, and female reproduction. As stated earlier, this view has a long Western philosophical history in the masculinist renditions of woman as soil, ground, incubator, and environment for man's seed. Man activates; woman grows the active material. As Judge Sorkow put it, "But for him, there would be no child."[79]

The California surrogate gestation decision treated reproduction on the male model. Law proceeds by analogy, and the analogue here is male. Gametes make the mom as they do the dad. A woman's parenthood in this case was decided on the same grounds as a man's parenthood—by virtue of her gamete contribution. Egg was equated to sperm, but sperm is still the standard. Nothing else mattered—not pregnancy, not labor, not the ongoing relationship between pregnant woman and fetus.

The egg acquires sperm status, however, only when it is not in conflict with the sperm. When "the egg" protests, as in the Whitehead-Stern case, she must fight for her rights and recognition. When "the egg" cooperates, as in the Johnson-Calvert case in which the egg was married to the sperm, the egg's rights are said to predominate. Unlike ejaculatory fathers, however, egg mothers can not win, unless conjoined with a male counterpart.

Privileging the "egg's rights," however, is just another form of essentialism, in which all reproduction is defined by the male standard. Eggs are to be treated like sperm; egg mothers like ejaculatory fathers. If men become legal fathers by virtue of sperm, women become legal mothers by virtue of eggs. The measurement of equality for women is being like men. In order to achieve rights, women must no longer prove that they are different from, as in the traditional legal calculus, but that they are the same as men.

Catharine MacKinnon has consistently exposed the fallacies of this sameness standard in law and legal theory: "Equality law tells women that they are entitled to equal treatment mainly to the degree they are the same as men. . . . The Court having since recognized that facial sex classifications [for example, statutory preferences given to men] may violate the equal protection clause, women were given the chance to meet the male standard in some cases." As women must now be equally considered for administrators of estates, eggs must also be considered as determinants of parenthood. "Women went from being categorically different to being putatively the same. . . . Having to be the same as men to be treated equally remains the standard."[80]

Since men are the standard, but men cannot (yet) become pregnant, pregnancy cannot be *the* determining element of parenthood. Such a pregnancy standard would deprive men of equal rights. Rather, women are recognized as parents to the extent that they do what men do, that is, generate eggs as men generate sperm. Women's parenthood is recognized only to the extent that it conforms to the legal determination of male parenthood and is "similarly situated," a legal phrase meaning measured by the same criteria. That a woman, as in the case of Anna Johnson, risks her health and well-being, undergoes nine months of pregnancy, and labors in birth is utterly devalued because it is not identical to the male reproductive act and experience. Confined by this analogy, women's more vital contributions to reproduction (pregnancy and birthing, personal and social relationship to the fetus becoming a child) are reduced to mere incubation, physical labor, and paid work in surrogacy. The significance of pregnancy, labor, and birth are shrunk to the size of sperm. Perhaps if and when new reproductive procedures give men the ability to become pregnant, pregnancy will become the determinant of parenthood!

Women are penalized for pregnancy. Equality in law is false, since the law does not recognize the real inequality that women face in law and in life for being pregnant, namely, male dominance and female subordination, not to mention the physical toll and debilitation that many women experience during pregnancy. The point is not a biological one; it is profoundly social with legal implications. Only women get pregnant, and only women are subjected to discrimination on these grounds. Especially in the context of surrogate gestation, women are specifically targeted for abuse because their pregnancies are perceived more negatively than usual. Not only is she pregnant, but she's pregnant "with someone else's child" who has no genetic link to her—for money.

Add to this that, in the Anna Johnson case, an African American woman was bearing a child for a white man and an Asian American woman. Radical feminists have long pointed out that surrogacy, especially surrogate gestation, invites the exploitation of Third World and minority women. Gena Corea predicted the Anna Johnson situation in 1985 when she warned that surrogate brokers and private individuals would seek out "authentic" surrogates—those who contribute no gametes—from indigent and cross-racial groups of women. With the development of surrogate gestation techniques, Corea predicted, the skin color would not matter.[81]

In surrogate gestation, however, there is an insidious way in which skin color does matter. It was not only Anna Johnson's lack of genetic connection that was used to argue against her in court. As writer Katha Pollitt has pointed out,

> It is safe to say that few American judges are going to take seriously the claims of a black woman to a nonblack child. Black women have, after all, always raised white children without acquiring any rights to them. Now they can breed them, too.[82]

Indeed, it appears that the Calverts may have selected Johnson precisely *because* her Black skin would ensure the Calverts' claim to the resultant child.

There have been no comparable public outcries or public debates about the Johnson-Calvert case as there were over the Whitehead-Stern case. Not many people seem concerned about its racist consequences or about its implications for an international market in surrogacy where women of color could easily be exploited and hired at a lower rate than the current market price of ten thousand U.S. dollars.

Nor have there been any public expressions of concern about the genetic essentialism established in this legal decision, which awards the child to the genetic parents. Those who worried mightily about the maternal essentialism they found inherent in privileging Mary Beth Whitehead's claim to the child seemingly have no similar concerns about the Anna Johnson case establishing a genetic entitlement to parenthood.

Following the California surrogate gestation decision, two genetic researchers at North Carolina State University were reported to have found that environmental conditions "in the womb of surrogate mothers may have long-lasting effects on their progeny."[83] It seems that research on mice indicates that the condition of the womb *does* affect fetal survival, birth weight, adult weight, bone structure, rate of growth, reproductive traits, and rate of early fat deposition and puberty. In summary, the experts have found evidence that "surrogate mother" mice *do* have an effect on how the fetus's genes get expressed, due to maternal-fetal interaction in the womb. In breeding dairy cows, for instance, the researchers tell us that "it is as important to use a good surrogate mother as to select an embryo with the desired milk-producing qualities."[84]

Having observed and tested the interactions of pregnant mice and their fetuses and armed with the evidence of breeding dairy cows, the experts confirmed the importance not of women, but of "the uterine environment." The relationship between a woman and her fetus is not real, that is, genetically influential, until men confirm that it is. When male experts present a "new" finding regarding maternal-fetal interaction, it is accepted. Yet women's experience, which established this "finding" long ago, has no independent validity without the confirmation of the male experts.

Expected Motherhood and Baby Craving

New reproductive technologies and contracts are on the rise at a time when the Western media are reminding women that if they reach thirty without having borne children, they are living half-lives. Since the ascendancy of the Reagan-Bush administrations in the United States and conservative and fundamentalist governments elsewhere, there has been a reemphasis on "family values" and the nuclear family. Two 1988 GOP presidential aspirants, Pat Robertson and Jack Kemp, brought the issue of low American fertility rates to the presidential campaign trail. In that same year, Pope John Paul II reaffirmed "the dignity of women" by prohibiting women from entering the priesthood but defended women's "equality" by stressing her vocation to motherhood. As the pope saw it, the "women's rights movement" poses a danger to women's dignity, because it encourages women to "appropriate to themselves male characteristics" and denies the nature of women as formed by maternal qualities.[85] The conservative religious and governmental climate has fostered both a withdrawal from political feminism and an emphasis on heterorelations.[86]

In Singapore, the birth rate has fallen below projected governmental figures. It has dwindled most among the "best and the brightest," and the government is especially taking note of the problem. Two-fifths of all women college graduates, if present trends continue, will not get married, and so Singapore will not have its "best and brightest" babies. Combine this with a population increase among Malays and Indians, and Singapore faces a supposed "birth dearth" of its dominant racial constituency.[87] Thus Singapore is embarking on the rapid development of new reproductive technologies. Concerned about the deficit of births among its educated elite, the government has opened the world's first egg bank. As the *International Herald Tribune* reported, "The major aim is to encourage career women, who tend to marry late, to have more children."[88]

The Birth Dearth is the title of a 1987 book authored by Ben Wattenberg of the conservative American Enterprise Institute. Its theme is that the "free, modern, industrial world" is not reproducing fast enough to replace itself and that there has not been enough of a decline in Third World fertility to stem the growth of its population. Women, that is, some women, are not bearing enough children over an extended period of time. As incomes rise, as women move into the work force, and as education increases, fertility falls. In an excerpt quoted from Wattenberg's book, the author writes,

> Demographer Charles Westoff of Princeton estimates that 50 percent of young American women will bear either no children or one child. . . .
>
> A study by Harvard and Yale social scientists described an America of the future with much depressed marriage rates. . . .
>
> Millions of young women were scared silly about the prospect of never marrying or having children. Yet somehow society seems to be directing them along that path.
>
> . . . Growing old without offspring is, quite simply, quite sad for most people.[89]

The Harvard-Yale study referred to by Wattenberg was one that the media touted as evidence that modern single women who had supposedly put career first were now realizing the error of their ways and craving marriage and motherhood. Since this study, the American media have been heavily promoting marriage and motherhood as necessary to the emotional well-being of the modern woman. The Harvard-Yale study was featured in widely read magazines such as *Newsweek* and *People*, which both gave it cover story prominence. According to the Harvard-Yale experts, a woman of thirty has a 20 percent chance of marrying; at thirty-five, her chances decrease to 5 percent; and at forty, *Newsweek* wrote that such upwardly mobile women were "more likely to be shot by a terrorist than ever to tie the knot."[90] The study, of course, depended on traditional heterorelational attitudes and perceptions such as women rushing "to catch husbands." That women might choose not to marry and have children, that women might find happiness, love, and security with other women, be they friends or lovers, was entirely precluded.[91]

Another article, from the late 1980s, featured on the front page of the *New York Times*, related the "sad stories" of a generation of "liberated" women, all single and approaching forty. The article was misrepresentatively titled "Single Women: Coping with a Void." In soap opera and wildly anecdotal style, Jane Gross wrote, "There is a single woman in New York, bright and accomplished, who dreads nightfall, when darkness hugs the city and lights go on in warm kitchens."[92] This article dredged up numerous examples of women who had "missed out" on marriage and kids. A closer examination of their narratives, however, reveals that the sad stories of these women were more the function of the reporter's interpretation and tone than of what was said by the women themselves. What the Harvard-Yale study and the *New York Times* article did not cite is the dismal marriage and family picture: the high incidence of child sexual and physical abuse, battered wives, the high divorce and remarriage rates, and the high increases in teenage pregnancy, which all challenge the picture of hearth and home as a haven for women and the site of total fulfillment. The *New York Times* reporter did observe that "women with less glamorous jobs seem to suffer far more," as well as women in "boring, day-to-day jobs," for whom "dating becomes important."[93] What these comments point to—in spite of what they are meant to convey—is the reality that many women are channeled into economically discriminatory, low-paying, deadended jobs that prompt them to seek material and emotional security in the traditional places—men, marriage, and family.

Many women might never have married and had children if such heterorelational, expected marriage, and pronatalist attitudes as expressed in the above sources had not impelled them. Motherhood as institution has compensated for a great deal of the oppression women experience inside and outside their homes. The media sentimentalize motherhood, along with the arrangements and technologies that make supposedly infertile women into mothers. The acceptance of motherhood and the sentimentalizing of female subordination has been women's stake in the system.

The assumption is that a woman is fulfilled through breeding. She enters reality only as a mother, and any woman who rejects that role is unnatural, suspect, and out of place. Various strategies are used to suggest and ultimately to ensure that women conform. The media portray women who do not marry and produce babies as living lives at the edge of despondency and despair. States use more hard-sell methods, for example, reversing liberal access to birth control and sanctioning the use of women as reproductive commodities. The media, the state, and other institutions manage motherhood and join together to try to crush the potential for independence in all women. The many subtle and not-so-subtle attacks on single women reflect this agenda, as do the various medical measures that have been instituted to manage women's reproductive capacities since the rise of gynecology and obstetrics in the nineteenth century. Motherhood as institution is meant to check female autonomy, to draw women back to the fold.

The political right has always used motherhood in a reactionary sense to glorify, disguise, and reinforce women's oppression. Its romanticizing of motherhood sentimentalizes women's subordination in the family as well as in society at large.

As women in various countries begin to confront issues of right-wing reproductive fundamentalism, sterilization abuse, contraception availability, and reproductive control, they find that the issue goes far beyond the use and abuse of specific reproductive technologies. Reproductive self-determination must be founded on women's achieving basic control in every area of their lives—most basically, the right and ability to choose *if* they want children, *when,* and *under what conditions.* Feminist advocacy of reproductive self-determination worldwide cannot merely point to the uses and abuses of the new reproductive technologies alone; it must advocate, as part of the content of such self-determination, the option to remain man-, marriage-, and child-free.

Feminism, however, will never challenge the compulsory nature of motherhood—motherhood as institution—until it challenges several other realities. It must confront the institutional context that directs women into marriage and/or motherhood while ignoring single and/or lesbian living as well as a child-free existence. It must encourage the latter options as *ways of living to be fostered,* not as lives to be tolerated and the less talked about, the better. Feminism has emphasized a woman's right to control her body in sexuality and reproduction. By emphasizing a woman's right to control her sexual and reproductive behavior, without acknowledging the possibility of opting out of heterosexuality and motherhood altogether, feminists have, by omission, supported prescriptive heterosexuality and motherhood.

White, Western, middle-class feminism has uncritically supported, as writer Judith Blake has pointed out, the "'do both' syndrome; i.e., motherhood and careers . . . as a combination to which all women have a right . . . thus stressing women's right not to have to make a choice."[94] As Martha Gimenez says, if childlessness were a legitimate option for women, it would have had as equally a prominent place as the "do both" syndrome in Western feminist writings.[95]

No technology of birth control or abortion, no amount of education about sexuality, no juggling of family roles to accommodate working mothers will ever give women control of their bodies and lives until women have the power to choose *not* to be wives and mothers and *not* to "do both." Reproductive self-determination means more than the technical means to ensure reproductive self-determination and voluntary childbearing. Until the option not to marry and not to have children is as encouraged and supported as traditional or alternative childbearing and -rearing, there is no real challenge to compulsory motherhood.

As a comprehensive political position, reproductive freedom must include a resistance to motherhood *as institution;* a refusal to profess loyalty to a system of subordination whose dynamic is the male control, use of, and access to women and what issues from women; and an affirmation of women's possibilities beyond motherhood and the metaphors of motherhood, that is, beyond nurturing, selfless giving, and caretaking the world. No emphasis on these moral qualities of women will free women, whether it comes from traditionalists such as Phyllis Schlafly who advocates that women "keep America good," or from feminists who want to affirm the differences that women have by virtue of their capacity to mother.

Motherhood is invariably portrayed as the material or metaphorical act for women's activity in the world. Thus other acts that women perform get relegated to a "reproductive consciousness"—acts such as peacemaking, nurturing, and creativity. All these activities are framed by the metaphors of motherhood and, in many instances, are seen to proceed from an innate biological capability, whether actualized or not. It is as if female peacemaking, nurturing, creativity, and ultimately the integrity and dignity of woman herself can be recognized and affirmed only in relation to her encompassing reproductive ability and consciousness.

The normative characterization of motherhood as women's true destiny will never change if women continue to accept female action in the world framed in maternal and reproductive metaphors. As the new reproductive technologies turn women into maternal environments and men into ejaculatory fathers, we must be wary of trying to right these wrongs by arguing for a new maternal essentialism, one that views motherhood as the source of women's power. Nor will women challenge the expanding definition of fatherhood with its concomitant political manifestation of father-right by reverting to motherhood as normative, instinctual, or the source of women's power. Women will never challenge the spermatic market—its surrogate stock and liquid assets—by idealizing motherhood as a collective power for women. Women's power does not come from a biological capacity. It proceeds from the collective courage and strength of women who, often under the worst of conditions, have claimed their power *as women who act in the world* and not in the service of men, and who have made that power work for other women.

CHAPTER THREE

A Critique of Reproductive Liberalism

Reproductive liberalism dominates the discourse and policy making of reproductive medicine in the United States and, increasingly, in other Western countries. Unlike reproductive conservatism, reproductive liberalism appears to be female-friendly. Like reproductive conservatism, however, it does little to ensure gender justice and is often antiwomen. Reproductive liberal-speak is not only the language of many progressives, but it is also prevalent in feminist writing on reproductive technologies and contracts.

Liberalism is, however, an ambiguous term. During politically conservative times, it becomes a synonym for radicalism and has been associated in public opinion with left-wing causes and ideologies. Thus liberal politicians shy away from publicly proclaiming the feared "L" word, as did Michael Dukakis during his 1988 presidential campaign. This causes others to wear the term as a badge of honor, as in the popular bumper sticker, "I'm a liberal and proud of it."

Reproductive liberalism, as represented by the reproductive technologies establishment of scientists, lawyers, policy makers, politicians, and academics, is actually a sort of reproductive fundamentalism. Its dominant principles, to be examined at length in this chapter, are: procreative liberty, gender neutrality, privacy, individual rights, and unlimited choice. I contend, however, that reproductive liberalism provides women with a supposed liberty that requires women to give up more freedom than we get; an individualistic inventory of reproductive rights in which almost anything can be claimed as a right; a gender-neutral theory and reality of rights and freedom; a concept of choice that is reduced to the option to consume; a right to privacy that is more accurately a right to private privilege for men (and some women) and that fosters a private enterprise in women's bodies; and a legal positivism separating rights from any substantive and ethical base of justice.

Procreative Liberty

Reproductive technologies and arrangements, such as surrogacy, have been affirmed as "procreative liberty." As promulgated by its major exponent, legal scholar John Robertson, procreative liberty is a fundamental right to reproduce that extends to the use of new reproductive technologies. Claiming that procreative liberty is grounded in the U.S. constitution, Robertson has popularized the concept and has been the chief legal missionary for promoting reproductive technologies and contracts based on this principle. He has developed a veritable thesaurus of phrases used in place of procreative liberty—"noncoital collaborative reproduction," "the right to use noncoital means," and "procreative autonomy."[1] Procreative liberty, in fact, has become a slogan of the new reproductive technologies establishment in much the same way that sexual freedom became the buzzword of the sexual liberation movement of the sixties.

U.S. arguments in favor of surrogacy illustrate the groundswell of reproductive liberal thinking based on procreative liberty. In the first New Jersey Superior court decision on the Baby M case in 1987, Judge Sorkow cited Robertson's interpretation of procreative liberty in his decision validating the surrogate contract. Referring to the arguments used by Bill Stern in defending the validity of the surrogate contract, Sorkow ruled, "The proponents of this surrogate parenting agreement argue that their right to enter such a contract is protected by a fundamental right to procreate. This right of procreation is bottomed in an individual's constitutional right of privacy secured by the 14th Amendment of the U.S. Constitution's substantive due process protections."[2]

Enumerating the legal precedents upholding this right to procreate, Sorkow reasoned that

> if one has a right to procreate coitally, then one has the right to reproduce non-coitally. . . . If it is reproduction that is protected, then the means of reproduction are also to be protected. . . . This court holds that the protected means extends to the use of surrogates.[3]

Quoting John Robertson's frequently cited article on procreative liberty (see note 1), Sorkow further stated, "It might even be argued that refusal to enforce these contracts and prohibition of money payments would constitute an unconstitutional interference with procreative liberty since it would prevent childless couples from obtaining the means with which to have families."[4]

This notion of procreative liberty claims to be based on the historical decisions rendered by U.S. courts that have avoided interfering in procreative decisions. In cases like *Griswold v. Connecticut* and *Roe v. Wade*, the courts have explicitly protected an individual's right *not to procreate*. Robertson contends that one can rightfully conclude from these cases that individuals have the correlative right *to procreate*. It is one thing, however, to legislate that an individual should not be forced to procreate against her will, and thereby protect legal access to contraception or abortion. It is quite another to derive from these legal protections the belief that individuals have the right to procreate by any means possible. There is no absolute right to procreate by any means possible, just as there is no absolute right to marry by any means possible. Individuals certainly have a right to marry, but there is no corresponding legal obligation for society to provide individuals with partners or with the means to meet a mate. If there are no legal provisions for the means to marry, why should there be legal provisions for the means to procreate?

Robertson leads a contingent of lawyers and scholars who advocate a virtually unlimited right to procreate by any means possible and who translate procreative liberty into the right to use any reproductive technology or arrangement. These procedures include surrogacy, IVF, sex predetermination, and genetic testing, among others.[5] The unarticulated agenda of the procreative liberty platform, however, is that *the right to use any reproductive procedure is actually the right to use any reproductive person.* When Robertson talks about the *means* of alternative reproduction, he refers to new reproductive contracts and procedures, but hidden in the discourse of means is the female person who is used. The undeclared reality is that *women are the means* to men's reproductive goals.

Robertson's notion of procreative liberty institutionalizes the commodification of women as means of procreation, and, in doing so, women become reproductive objects and instruments for others' ends. Procreative liberty also institutionalizes children as products who are quality controlled by an array of reproductive technologies and arrangements. Robertson is not defending a simple, well-meaning desire for children. Rather, his version of procreative liberty is rooted in the quest for children who are technologically and contractually vetted, "made to order" in accordance with genetic, gender, racial, and physical characteristics that are determined and selected mostly by men.

It is not enough to say that infertile people should be able to realize their reproductive goals and that this is a good to be unconditionally promoted by any means. The assumption that any reproductive means should be a constitutionally protected procreative liberty ignores the real means used to bring about the desired end. Procreative liberty is not an abstract end, separate from an evaluation of the means. The central fact is that women's bodies are the reproductive means to others' reproductive goals.

Robertson's version of procreative liberty treats procreation and its technological procedures as ends in isolation from any other consideration—the nature of the reproductive arrangement, the exploitation of the women involved, and the way in which these reproductive procedures will immediately and ultimately affect the value and status of all women in a gender-based society. Procreative liberty as defined by the reproductive liberals increases women's reproductive exploitation, not women's reproductive independence.

Gender-Neutral Equality Equals Inequality for Women

Procreative liberty is supposedly a gender-neutral right. Gender neutrality pretends to be gender equality premised on an already established parity between women and men. The use of the rhetoric of equality, however, hides women's actual inequality and the privileging of men's reproductive goals. The promotion of gender-neutral rights obscures the real privilege and dominance of men.

Many proponents of the new reproductive techniques have compared surrogacy to artificial insemination, arguing that if men can sell sperm, women should be able to sell their uterine capacities. At the very least, this is a grossly distorted symmetry. Contractual procreation in surrogacy amounts to the total use of a woman's person for nine months. "Popping sperm" is hardly the equivalent of "popping a baby," as the equalizers imply. Additionally, as surrogacy is used with other reproductive technologies such as in vitro fertilization, sex predetermination, and super-ovulation, the so-called surrogate must also submit herself to a series of invasive and often debilitating procedures devised to ensure that she get pregnant quicker and produce a contractually designed baby.

Gender equality amounts to an abstract right when the real conditions of women's inequality are glossed over and not given legal weight. In the area of custody, for example, we see that the courts increasingly award more and more fathers custody of their children *when fathers decide to fight for custody* because, for one thing, the real inequality of women's economic and social situation is made invisible.[6] What women come to court *without* versus what men arrive in court *with* gets no legal recognition. The law presumes that everything is equal at the judicial starting line. In fact, however, the father is most often in an economically advantaged situation and has typically made a second marriage. So-called equality within a gender-neutral context, as in this custody example, where all things are presumed to be equal, thus gets turned into a political and legal weapon against women and serves to bolster father-right.

In surrogacy disputes, the far greater legal and financial resources of the "ejaculatory father"—the middle-class home, education, and upbringing that he can provide—measured against the usual financially disadvantaged position of the so-called surrogate mother and her often insecure family situation privileges the sperm source immediately in any court battle, as happened in the Baby M case. The liberal principle of equality thus results in an actual inequality for women as evidenced in the results of surrogacy disputes, where the contracting male has won most of these cases.

We cannot assume that anything, be it surrogacy or no-fault divorce, will promote women's equality unless we first admit the conditions of women's inequality and male dominance in which surrogacy and divorce disputes are located. Worldwide, the situation of women is appalling, but U.S. statistics alone provide a sobering view and dose of reality. Full-time white women workers earn 64.7 percent of what white men earn, but 30 percent of employed women work part-time. African American women earn 60.3 percent while Latina women earn 54.6 percent of what white men earn. Women receive much lower benefits from Social Security because most work in low-paying, high-turnover jobs and leave the job market to bear and rear children and care for sick or elderly relatives. Of all eleven million AFDC (Aid for Families with Dependent Children, "welfare") recipients, 94 percent are women and children. An estimated 25 percent of women have experienced an unwanted sexual encounter with a male adult before age thirteen; 87 percent of child sexual assaults are female; 42 to 90 percent of employed women experience sexual harassment, depending on how sexual harassment is defined; the feminist network of rape crisis centers estimates that one out of every three women will be raped; and a Presidential Task Force estimates that 50 to 70 percent of wives experience battery during their marriages.[7] These are but a few of the real "equality" statistics. It is, therefore, an understatement to maintain that any substantive concept of legal equality must recognize that women cannot move from inequality to equality without a *real, material* recognition of the conditions of male dominance within which women make legal claims.

Most so-called surrogates arrive in court from a background of economic disadvantage or dead-endedness. The public portrays them as unfit and unnatural mothers in a society where a primary role of women has been as breeders, and men are privileged by a history of male entitlement to women and children. These are not mere gender differences between women and men, where the presumed legal starting line is that all things are equal. A legal recognition of male dominance, thus a legal recognition of the ways in which women have been channeled into surrogacy and motherhood at any cost to themselves, is a necessary legal precondition to women's equality. Rights are related to actual social relations, and it is male-dominant relations that are definitive in the legal area—the man's relation to his sperm, his money, his wife, and the women who may serve as surrogate wives, that is, as surrogate breeders.

Rights are by definition rights *to* something given in the present social order. Rights are often framed in terms of individual or group access to a prevailing social order without challenging the social relations inherent in that structure. The right to equality, the right to procreate, and even the right to choose what to do with one's own body fail to address the underlying structure of male-dominant social relations in which certain women are created as a breeder class and where women are commodified as reproductive beings to be bought and sold in the spermatic marketplace.

Privacy

Closely allied with the gender-neutral principles of procreative liberty and equality is the gender-neutral notion of *privacy*. The right to privacy is always invoked by the defenders of the new reproductive technologies and can be summed up in the words of surrogacy advocate Lori Andrews: "The constitutional right to privacy protects procreative autonomy. As state courts have recognized, the right to privacy to make procreative decisions sets the context for recognizing the right to use a surrogate mother."[8] Thus so-called procreative liberty is grounded in the constitutional right to privacy. The right to privacy has allowed the abuse of women in many spheres—domestic, sexual, and reproductive. A woman's right to privacy often translates into a man's right to do with/to her what he wishes, shrouded in the privacy of his bedroom, his courts, and his country.

The defense of abortion rights in the United States has been built on the right of privacy, and *Roe v. Wade* has rested on this legal pillar. Over the last fifteen years, however, some feminists have maintained that Roe's gender neutrality is its primary legal liability to women and one of the reasons why it has been gradually eroded—the fact that it is not grounded in any tradition of *women's* civil rights. Nevertheless, alternative reproductive arrangements continue to be grounded in the right to privacy.

This right to privacy, however, is a right to private male privilege, where women remain the private property of men and male-dominant private enterprise. As private privilege, surrogacy actually protects the private reproductive desires of the male sperm source by legitimating the leasing of a woman's body to be used as his private procreative property. As private enterprise, the surrogate agencies provide the means by which the right to procreate can be exercised in private, with all discretion, unless the breeder-property reneges on her contract and goes public. In reality, the right to privacy favors the proprietary and professional claims of the "ejaculatory fathers" and the brokerage agencies.

The right to privacy has moved from the sexual to the reproductive sphere, from the bedrooms of supposedly consenting adults to the boardrooms of surrogate brokerage agencies and medical entrepreneurs who now demand contractual "consent" of women used as surrogates. From a man's private entitlement to a woman's body in prostitution and pornography, the right to privacy includes yet another private male entitlement—his access to her reproductive capacities. Because these capacities are defined as sexual and reproductive, which have been traditionally relegated to the personal sphere, they are therefore deemed private. Any limitations on sexuality and reproduction thus become limitations on privacy rather than legal protections for women.

There is a lot more at stake in sexuality and reproduction than any one individual's right to procreate. There is a lot more at stake than the right to procreate of any *group,* for example, those who are infertile or those who want children through alternative reproductive means. These so-called rights may benefit some individual women, but more often they benefit individual men and men as a class. In the long run, they diminish the individual and social rights of all women and ignore the impact of these techniques on the status of women worldwide.

Pro-Choice, Abortion, and Technological Reproduction

Pro-choice has become the rallying cry of women's and reproductive rights groups in the United States today. Not pro-woman, but pro-choice, as if the latter might attract those who are not certain about their commitment to women's rights but are indeed committed to the quintessential American value of choice. Reliance on choice, especially as promoted by women's groups, lacks not only vision but honesty.

Pro-choice lingo escalated in the aftermath of the 1989 U.S. Supreme Court decision effectively giving states broader authority to limit abortions (*Webster v. Reproductive Services*). In the wake of this legal carnage, women's and reproductive rights groups formed coalitions and intensified their promotion of choice. The language of choice, rather than the language of women's rights, was reinforced as the ideological weapon aimed at anti-abortion fundamentalism. Appeals for reproductive rights have been voiced almost entirely in the language of choice.

Technological and contractual reproduction has also been defended as reproductive choice. Reproductive liberals have linked new reproductive arrangements and technologies with abortion, arguing that both must be defended if reproductive choice is to be preserved for women, equating the protection of technological reproduction with the protection of abortion. Over the last five years especially, many pro-choice advocates have emphasized that people of conscience must support new reproductive arrangements such as embryo freezing, IVF, and surrogacy, arguing for expanded access to these procedures not only for infertile women and men, but also for single and lesbian women, single and homosexual men, and various minority and economically disadvantaged groups.

The reproductive liberals—the technologists and doctors, the surrogate brokers, the lawyers—have been adept at manipulating pro-choice philosophy and politics, knowing that many will accept the rhetoric without questioning the reality of what is promoted as choice. The American Fertility Society, in its report outlining ethical and legal justifications for the use of alternative reproductive procedures, not only stacked its committee with reproductive liberals but used the language of choice and procreative liberty to promote all the new reproductive arrangements under consideration. The report's initial section, which outlines the basis for evaluating an ethical position, is grounded in "The Constitutional Aspects of Procreative Liberty." In the following section, entitled "American Law and the New Reproductive Technologies," the committee asserts, "In a country that gives to childbearing decisions a legal protection of magnitude unparalleled in the rest of the world, *professional guidelines must not casually accede to restrictions on reproductive technologies that offer enhanced options.*"[9] Heralded as "enhanced options" *before* it is demonstrated that they offer enhanced options, new reproductive procedures are blessed immediately.

To be pro-choice, however, is *not* necessarily to be pro-woman. Gary Skoloff, the lawyer for Bill Stern in the first Baby M trial, argued that if the court failed to uphold the surrogate contract, women who wanted to become surrogates would be deprived of their right to choose. Here choice is more rhetoric than reality, a superficial slogan exploited by surrogate lawyers and brokers, in which women are accorded the right to choose surrogacy with all the eloquence never voiced on behalf of women's right to earn, for example, the same money that men earn.

It is time to examine what choices men, and some women, defend as our right and what choices these same men and women will not defend as our right. Why is women's right to choose surrogacy widely defended at the same time that women's more substantive human, civil, and economic rights are being suppressed, at the same time that affirmative action is being gutted, and at the same time that there is still no Equal Rights Amendment to the Constitution? The choice to become a surrogate is hardly the freedom for which most women have been fighting.

The Banalizing of Choice: Choice as Consumption

Choice is increasingly allied with consumption in contemporary society; the right to choose has effectively become the right to consume. For years, corporate America has collapsed choice and consumption to sell questionable products. In 1978, a spokesman for Upjohn, manufacturer of Depo-Provera, opposed FDA regulation of contraceptives on the grounds that it deprived the public of "free choice." What he did not articulate was that regulation deprived the company of its "right" to manufacture what it wanted, and it deprived the public of its "right" to consume what the company deemed its range of choices/commodities. In 1989, R. J. Reynolds was attacked for targeting women with its new brand of cigarettes, through ads intended to appeal especially to females. The company's vice president responded by stating that he believed women to be just as capable as men of making an adult choice. And in 1992, as the numbers of silicone breast implant mutilations were being revealed to the FDA and the public, Dow-Corning continued to defend the implants as the right choice for many women. In fact, the rhetoric of choice has been central to the marketing of many questionable and dangerous products.

Professional and corporate so-called consumer advocates are often influential in convincing the potential buyer that she or he needs to consume a particular product. Citing consumer demand, the corporate and professional reproductive technology advocates are now promoting alternative reproductive procedures such as IVF and surrogacy as commodities. These commodities, however, are available only to the few—usually white, middle class, heterosexual, and able bodied.

Choice as consumerism has few limits. Limits, within the liberal expansionism of technological reproduction, are regarded as repressive; to limit is to repress choice. From an environmental perspective, however, the lack of limits is disastrous (see chapter 4). The physical exploitation of the environment continues, in part, because there is a total indifference to any kind of limits—limits that are necessary if nature is to survive. Likewise, the reproductive exploitation of women continues because there have been few limits to medical-technical expansionism promoted as choice. The new reproductive technologies are at the center of the exponential medicalization of women's bodies.

Represented as expanding women's choice, IVF technology, for example, actually narrows the life choices of women who consume this technology. The testimony of many women who have gone through the IVF treadmill, returning again and again to a clinic for the hoped-for child, is not a glowing confirmation of expanded life choices for women.

> This is the forty-seventh time I have felt hope slipping out of me in a relentless stream of menstrual discharge. I know it is the forty-seventh time because my computer tells me so. The crisp, cool headings displayed on the monitor were designed to make me feel more in control: "Number of days in cycle," "Days of intercourse during fertile period," "Test performed." Instead, I feel my life spinning away from me while I obligingly record the symptoms.
>
> . . . I have never before taken seriously the idea of giving up. You see, giving up, for the infertile, is not really an option at all. We make our reproductive decisions as members of a society that believes a woman's primary function is motherhood. . . . We see this reinforced constantly in television commercials, in designer baby clothes stores, in our Christmas traditions, in our parents' pointed questions, in families strolling through the park. . . .

. . . The pursuit of motherhood take[s] over our lives because so much—self-identity, self-esteem, self-image—depends on it. . . .

. . . P.S. After more than four years of infertility, I am pregnant. . . . The last three months have been a black hole of terror. The overwhelming fatigue and constant nausea were bad enough, but the fear of miscarriage nearly drove me crazy. . . . I have done nothing for three months but brood, sleep and feel sick. . . . I live from one obstetrical appointment to the next.[10]

Women must take a hard look at what is offered to us as choice. The items available in the new reproductive supermarket are arranged by medical-technical interests, often in concert with other professional middlemen. Traditionally, as ethicist Beverly Wildung Harrison has written,

> *Choice* in a medical context usually is construed as an individual "case" problem and treated as an issue of professional discernment. Doctors and other health-care professionals frequently view social reality as external to a technical medical context and biological considerations as abstractable from the deeper social setting. This strongly reinforces the "discrete-deed" approach. . . .[11]

This is true, but it is too benevolent an analysis, as if only the history of medical training prompts an individualist calculus of a problem. Harrison does not account for the fact that doctors transform the "discrete deed" into a patient's personal need. We must examine how an "individual case problem," for example, infertility, is made into a technical option, for example, IVF, surrogacy, or embryo transfer and freezing. Prior to consumer demand, there are potent professional and commercial interests involved in the development and proliferation of these techniques. The reproductive choices presented are the medical-technical options made available. The right to choose has become merged with the right of the technological progenitors not to have their offerings questioned.

Options always grow out of contexts. In vitro fertilization emerges from a medical context primed for technical developments and research ambitions. This context fades into the background, though, as researchers, clinicians, and the media instead highlight the desperation of individuals who want children. Surrogacy grows out of a context of female subordination, poverty, and the relegation of women to their supposedly legitimate work, that is, breeding. The ease with which the right to choose shrinks to the right to consume should make us examine carefully the consumer-designed context of the new reproductive supermarket.

Reproductive Liberalism Defined as Feminism

Reproductive liberalism underlies the work of a number of feminist proponents of surrogacy and technological reproduction. Much of the feminist advocacy of new reproductive arrangements has come from women who, in former times, might have been described as socialist feminists. More recently, however, much of their writing is more accurately described as postmodernist in theme and theory. I choose to describe them as reproductive liberals since, as with reproductive liberals in general, they endorse procreative liberty, gender neutrality, privacy, unlimited choice, and the promotion of the so-called liberating facets of reproductive technology for women.

Historically, many socialist feminists have espoused sexual liberalism. As Sheila Jeffreys has shown, socialist feminists advocated classic liberal positions during the nineteenth and twentieth centuries when they opposed the work of early radical feminists fighting against sexual assault, prostitution, and sexual slavery.[12] More recently, some socialist feminists have promoted sexual liberalism, drawing from positions that permeated nineteenth- and twentieth-century socialist feminism.[13] Over the last decade, socialist feminists have joined with other academic and professional sexual liberals to oppose the feminist antipornography campaign and have broadened their views to affirm sadomasochistic sexuality, man-boy "love," and prostitution.

We are now witnessing a liberalism that defines itself as feminism in the reproductive realm. This liberalism has opposed itself to the feminist resistance against new reproductive technologies and contracts. Like its sexual counterpart, which promoted male-dominant modes of sexuality as sexual liberation, feminist reproductive liberalism affirms surrogacy, in vitro fertilization, and many new reproductive procedures as reproductive freedom for women.

Feminist analysis and activism against the new reproductive technologies burgeoned in the early 1980s. Recognizing that technological developments were rapidly escalating on an international scale, women from First and Third World countries came together in 1984 to share information, shape analysis and response, and specifically name how these technologies harmed women. The challenge to this gathering of international feminists was to reorient the ethical and political discussion from a fetus-centered and gender-neutral view to a woman-centered perspective. That reorientation was largely due to the efforts and activism of FINRRAGE members.[14]

In the mid 1980s, however, another brand of feminist analysis of the new reproductive technologies took shape, emanating from the United States and, later, from Britain. It advanced a more "nuanced" and "sophisticated" assessment of these technologies, arguing that women could use them with benefit (while being abused by them). Some of this justification initially appeared in sections of the *Reproductive Laws for the 1990s: A Briefing Handbook* associated with the Women's Rights Litigation Project at Rutgers University and in Michelle Stanworth's volume, *Reproductive Technologies.*[15]

Reproductive liberalism is much broader and more powerful than its feminist version. But it is important to examine the feminist liberal arguments advocating new reproductive procedures as a woman's choice, because reproductive liberals, especially in the United States and Britain, are seen as representing *the* feminist position on technological and contractual reproduction. Because of their institutional and professional hegemony, the so-called feminist debates about the new reproductive technologies in the United States are managed by the feminist reproductive liberals since it is they who dominate women's studies programs, the feminist media and journals, and the women's research institutes, and they serve as evaluators to granting agencies. Effectively, they have become the gatekeepers of feminist knowledge, presenting a more radical feminist politics as flawed and extremist. It is therefore important that feminist reproductive liberalism be critiqued and that radical feminism speak for itself.

1. The Balancing Act

Feminist reproductive liberals give priority to the question—which begs its answer—how do these technologies benefit women? This in itself is a peculiar chronology of inquiry since, one would assume, before deciding that such technologies *can* benefit women, one would have to prove the case. Yet the agenda is always framed by this initial question/answer. And following from this initial question/answer, a second one: how do "we" ensure equal access to the technologies for everyone—poor, Black, and lesbian women, for example? Editor Michelle Stanworth, in the introductory essay to *Reproductive Technologies,* asks "whether we can create the political and cultural conditions in which such technologies can be employed by women to shape the experience of reproduction according to their own definitions."[16]

Hilary Rose also argues that "the IVF cat is out of the bag, and—whatever else IVF does—it meets real needs for (some) real women. Consequently a feminism that accepts the diversity of women's needs must now work to limit IVF's imperialistic claims over women's bodies, and its associated claim to consume even more of the health-care budget for high-tech, curative medicine."[17] While pointing to the technological hegemony, nonetheless Rose seems to believe that IVF can be made available for some while restricting it for the many, in the interests of limiting high-tech and high-budget medicine.

As early as 1970, Shulamith Firestone suggested some supposed benefits of new reproductive technologies in *The Dialectic of Sex.*[18] But she was page-lashed ruthlessly as naively optimistic by some of the same feminists who are now urging us to take a more balanced view of these technologies. As they critique much radical feminist writing, so they depicted Firestone's work as offering only facile solutions. In other words, she did not perform the recent balancing act of being *both for and against.* Having it both ways, in effect, sums up the more "nuanced" reproductive liberal critique. It poses as a sophisticated rational approach to both sides of the issue, encouraging women to recognize how these technologies not only abuse women but also how they can be used in women's own interests. Like the ways in which pain has been equated with pleasure for women, so too is abuse fused with use.

2. *The Ontological Argument: All Radical Feminists Are Essentialists*

Much of the feminist reproductive liberal critique caricatures radical feminist arguments against the technologies. Reproductive liberals fault critics of the new reproductive technologies for making motherhood naturalistic, biologistic, and almost atavistic—as radical feminism itself has been typed as essentialist and ontological. A mythical state of natural motherhood is conjured up from nowhere so that feminists who oppose technological and contractual reproduction can be attacked as dragging women back to the days of "anatomy is destiny" and as pitting nature against technology. For example, Michelle Stanworth cautions that "the attempt to reclaim motherhood as a female accomplishment should not mean giving the natural priority over the technological—that pregnancy is natural and good, technology unnatural and bad."[19]

Radical feminist opponents of the new reproductive technologies do not pit nature against technology, nor do we extol a new version of biology is destiny for women. Opposition to these technologies is based on the more political feminist perspective that *women as a class have a stake in reclaiming the female body, not as female nature, but by refusing to yield control of it to men, to the fetus, to the state, and most recently to those liberals who advocate that women control our bodies by giving up control.*

Reducing radical feminism to the term *cultural feminism,* which they then set out to disparage, Juliette Zipper and Selma Sevenhuijsen blame cultural feminists, especially in the United States, for returning women to "nurturance, naturalness and love" and for extolling "natural motherhood and natural procreation" as "the real values of feminism."[20] They assert that feminist analysis must "shake free from the ideological inheritance of cultural feminism" and especially from the presupposition that the mother-child bond is sacrosanct.[21] Much of their criticism, however, is an artifact beginning with the term *cultural feminism.* As elaborated by Alice Echols, cultural feminism defines a potpourri of radical feminist simplifications, reductionisms, and distortions that run the gamut from invoking "biological explanations of gender differences" to a vilification of the left![22] Lynne Segal serves up a British variant on this theme of critiquing radical feminism as cultural feminism in her book, *Is the Future Female?* "Mostly from North America, where it is known as 'cultural feminism,' it celebrates women's superior virtue and spirituality and decries 'male' violence and technology. . . . Feminists . . . like me recall that we joined the women's movement to challenge the myths of women's special nature."[23]

Both Echols and Segal, for the most part, ignore the radical feminist critique of biological determinism and consistent emphasis on the social and political construction of women's lives. They quote selectively from radical feminist authors who have specified at great length and in great detail our own critiques of biological determinism and female essentialism, yet nowhere do they acknowledge these critiques. As feminist activist and writer Liz Kelly notes, the critique of biological determinism is one of the things that many radical and socialist feminists have always held in common. However, especially in their theories of sexuality, many socialist feminists ignore the dominant tendency in their own accounts of female and male socialization, which "are far more essentialist than their radical feminist counterparts. By drawing on revised Freudian categories, they offer a much more determined and limited view of change."[24]

As with sexuality, so too with reproduction. Liberal feminist writings on the new reproductive technologies portray women—especially women who are infertile—as *needing* these technologies. This conforms to the rationale of the medical and technological progenitors who constantly present these technologies as fulfilling the desperate needs of infertile women—not the researchers' own desperate needs for scientific advancement, status, and financial gain.

Feminists who oppose technological and contractual reproduction have recognized that motherhood is depicted increasingly as a *need* for women. Radical feminist opponents of the technologies have been extremely critical of the ways doctors and the media fit these technologies into *their* proposed vision of women's supposed natural motherhood and the ways in which women are channeled into trying yet one more invasive and debilitating medical procedure in order to become pregnant. Yet every time radical feminists cite the myth and manipulation of maternity—the revival of natural motherhood—by the medical and scientific progenitors, it is we who are faulted for perpetuating a naturalistic view of motherhood.

3. The "How Dare We Define Feminism" Approach

In a 1988 review of *Made to Order*, an anthology of writing opposed to new reproductive technologies, appearing in *The Women's Review of Books*,[25] Rayna Rapp criticizes the book for equating "feminism with opposition to the new reproductive technologies, as if there were a unified category called 'woman' whose natural ability to bear children now stands under the threat of total male, mechanical medical take-over. . . . Labelling a single oppositional stance as 'feminist' and anything else as 'not' prematurely forecloses the strategies we need to develop."[26] The equation is Rapp's, not that of the authors in *Made to Order*. But beyond this false equation is another more troubling concern.

"Don't call your position feminist" has become one of the ten commandments of sexual and reproductive liberalism. This convoluted prohibition effectively says that feminists cannot dare to articulate what feminism means because if we do we are mouthing a single, correct-line, exclusionary feminist position. Articulating what feminism means, however, seems not exclusionary but honest. If we do not articulate what feminism means, what does feminism mean? And then we can debate what feminism means, rather than how dare we think we can say what feminism means!

It would be much more fruitful to talk about the issues and the content of our differing positions than about relative postures of authority. The authority that anyone asserts in defining a position that is for or against or somewhere on the so-called more nuanced spectrum should come from an informed and reflective assessment, as well as her belief in the rightness of what she is saying. We must all take responsibility for our positions and argue the issues.

4. The Accusations of Absolutism Approach

Increasingly, *opposition* is translated as absolutism. *Absolutism* is an overused word to discredit the position of those who take a strong and often passionate stand. For example, Rebecca Albury in *Australian Feminist Studies* attacks, among other things, the position of well-known Australian feminist critic Robyn Rowland: "Rowland has tended to enter the public debate with an absolutist moral position. . . ."[27]

An oppositional stance is out of fashion in feminism, as is outrage, passion, and explicit political activism. Radical feminist writing is derided as reading "like a communique from the front lines."[28] Of course, one very well may be on the front lines, but that seems negligible. There was a time in this wave of feminism when it was honorable—not a cause for dismissal—to be on the front lines.

Many German FINRRAGE members experienced these front lines during the 1987 staging of thirty-three simultaneous raids by the Bundeskriminalamt (the German equivalent of the FBI) in the then West Germany. Files, research, radio and video recordings, address lists, and personal documents were seized by heavily armed police (two hundred in Essen alone), and during the raids women were forced to undress in order for police to note "non-changeable marks" on their bodies for future reference. Two women were jailed and one was kept in solitary confinement for two years, charged under the terrorist act.[29] The raids were directed overwhelmingly against feminist critics of genetic and reproductive technology.

Consistently, radical feminist critics of surrogacy and technological reproduction are faulted for their "absolutist" and oppositional approach and their failure to ask the "more complex" question of under what conditions the new reproductive technologies might be useful to women. Rosalind Petchesky, for example, cautions feminist critics of the new reproductive technologies to recognize "complex elements" [that] cannot easily be generalized or, unfortunately, vested with privileged insight."[30] Terms like *absolutist, totalizing, universal* conjure up images of simplemindedness and a lack of thinking on the part of those who oppose the new reproductive technologies. Supposedly, those who do more tough-minded thinking would emerge with a more balanced position. And presumably, those who are more attentive to race, culture, sexuality, and class will always take a provisional position on any women's issue. This critique is applied by liberals to *women's* issues but not, for instance, to progressive Central American or South African politics. If one is not a moral relativist on women's issues, one is by definition an absolutist.

Since the 1970s, socialist feminists have been accusing radical feminists of not having a class and cross-cultural analysis. They have consistently plied this line even in the face of evidence to the contrary. When the evidence could no longer be ignored, then the rhetoric changed. Radical feminists did not have the "right kind" of class and/or cross-cultural analysis. For example, Rayna Rapp also attacks *Made to Order* for "simply asserting solidarity with third world women and including essays that portray their condition."[31] Being unable to chastise the collection for *not* including a cross-cultural analysis, she now finds the analysis *merely* "included." This is a patronizing and arrogant assumption; the essays of women from Brazil and Bangladesh are not "simply" included. They are an integral part of the analysis of the book, which offers an international spectrum of essays by women from France, Germany, Australia, the United States, England, Switzerland, and the Netherlands. Rapp's logic is all the more incongruous given her enthusiastic praise for the second volume under review, *Reproductive Technologies*, which is almost completely authored by Anglo and U.S. women and includes little international analysis and no Third World perspective.

Academic and professional feminism in the United States today is permeated by sexual and reproductive liberalism, not by sexual and reproductive radicalism. Fortunately, feminism outside the academy and the professions is much more radical and vibrant. U.S. sexual and reproductive liberalism has been narrowly focused on individual "rights," "needs," and "desires." In the surrogacy context, for example, the constant talk about rights has deceived many U.S. women into thinking that we have more rights than we actually possess. One thing that I have found refreshing about working in an international context is that women from other countries, particularly in the developing world, have no illusions about their so-called rights.

Feminist liberalism has transformed women's reproductive abuse in technological and contractual reproduction into women's reproductive need, in the same way that the sexual liberals reconstructed the sexual abuse of women in pornography, prostitution, and sadomasochistic sexuality as women's sexual pleasure. There are also, however, important differences between sexual and reproductive liberal feminists. In feminist reproductive liberal circles, there is more opposition to surrogacy and more criticism of technological reproduction than was ever expressed about pornography.

One reason for this may be a visceral female identification with motherhood and children and with the importance of preserving this realm from abuse. Additionally, reproductive issues are seen as the domain of women, something women have the right to defend, especially in the name of children, whereas freedom from sexual abuse is something that women have to defend in their own name. Thus reproductive freedom is perceived as a broader issue that affects not only women, but children and men as well. It is not so singly identifiable as a woman's issue.

More instrumental has been the male history of support for reproductive rights. This comes especially from leftist and liberal men who have aligned themselves with campaigns for women's reproductive freedom, perceiving that their own interests are very much at stake. For example, *Playboy* magazine has consistently funded pro-choice abortion projects and supported pro-choice policy and legislation because it is in the best interests of progressively political, upwardly mobile men—playboys—not to be encumbered with the consequences of heterosex.

> It was the brake that pregnancy put on fucking that made abortion a high-priority political issue for men in the 1960s.... The decriminalization of abortion—for that was the political goal—was seen as the final fillip: it would make women absolutely accessible, absolutely "free." The sexual revolution, in order to work, required that abortion be available to women on demand. If it were not, fucking would not be available to men on demand.... The male-dominated Left agitated for and fought for and argued for and even organized for and even provided political and economic resources for abortion rights for women. The Left was militant on the issue.[32]

Many so-called enlightened men promote reproductive rights for women, especially in areas such as contraception and abortion, whereas there is little male support for antipornography politics. Rather, the liberal establishment tries to malign women as prudes and puritans when they attack the sexual politics of a male-dominant culture. Liberals have also sought to discredit antipornography feminists by allying them with the politics of the right wing.

It appears far easier for feminist liberals to embrace reproductive freedom than to advocate for women's sexual freedom *from* the male-dominant modes of sexuality such as prostitution and pornography. Instead, liberals embrace women's sexual freedom *for* the male-dominant modes of sexuality. Their version of sexual freedom equals sexual pleasure, bracketed from any critique of women's sexual abuse.

Because many of the feminist reproductive liberals come from a socialist feminist background, they have regarded reproductive politics as more their terrain than sexual politics. Radical feminists have been more closely allied with issues of pornography, rape, sexual harassment, sexual abuse, woman battering, and other areas of sexual objectification and violence than have socialist feminists. The consistent historical tension between radical feminists and socialist feminists around issues of sexual abuse, dating back to the beginnings of this century, may provide one reason why some socialist feminists have taken a *political* stand against surrogacy and not against pornography.

Other socialist feminists, however, have come out in support of surrogacy. They uphold the liberal wedge argument that state interference with any so-called reproductive right will allow state repression of those few limited reproductive gains that women have won, mostly in the areas of contraception and abortion. Thus they find themselves in the position of having to play off one so-called reproductive right (the right to procreate by any means possible) against another—the right not to procreate (abortion). And they see any legal prohibitions on surrogacy as endangering the right to abortion. Furthermore, they subscribe to a superficial reasoning that the man's claim to the child is equal to the woman's. Accordingly, they argue that privileging the woman's claim is reverting to special protectionism that is reactionary toward women and fosters a maternal essentialism based upon a regressive notion of biological mother-right.

Socialist feminism has historically avoided the radical feminist emphasis on addressing how men—not only social or economic systems—oppress women. It has chosen to frame women's oppression largely in economic terms and has shunned any consistent analysis of sexuality as *male-dominant power.* Thus it pays little serious attention to how so-called normal sexuality depends on women's oppression, since sexuality is not recognized as a male-dominant system in and of itself. For example, socialist feminist studies of women in the workplace have historically documented women's oppression through health hazards and economically dead-ended work, with little mention of sexual harassment as affecting women's work performance.

Socialist feminists, with few exceptions, have not put much premium on the sexual abuse of women in pornography, prostitution, and the male-dominant modes of sexuality. Instead, their politics of sexuality reduces to a politics of desire magically sprung free from male sexual domination and abuse, a classic theme of laissez-faire liberalism. Their tendency has been to see any campaign against sexual abuse, pornography, and the male power modes of sexuality as a sideline, as a distraction from women's real oppression, whatever that may be, and indeed as a reactionary trap for women, equated with a conservative movement for social purity.[33]

Further, socialist feminist critique of reproductive abuses has taken little note of the *connections* between the reproductive abuse of women and women's sexual oppression. Their reproductive politics has no sexual political foundation. For example, socialist feminists have focused on issues such as sterilization abuse, abortion rights, economic provisions for working mothers such as childcare, and access to birth control for more women, without wanting to recognize that more is at stake. They have emphasized *reproductive rights* and *reproductive access* for women to birth control and abortion and now, by extension, to the new reproductive technologies. But they include no analysis of women's access to an independent sexuality freed from male definition and desire.

When a substantive reproductive freedom is not joined with a substantive sexual freedom, as it is not in a traditional socialist feminist calculus of reproductive rights, the result is a reproductive liberalism. The insistent refusal of many socialist feminists to admit the central importance of a radical feminist critique of the male power modes of sexuality is largely responsible for this liberalism and for the lack of connection between sexuality and reproduction.

Surrogacy's availability is the result of the conditions men establish among themselves to grant access to women and women's reproductive capacities. A critique of surrogacy that remains fixated at the level of providing workable economic options for women in the surrogate industry and tightening up the contract so as to remove some of the more extreme abuses to women never addresses the nature of surrogacy within the total context of the male access to women. Reproductive liberalism offers women no substantive vision of reproductive freedom or rights.

Women as Victims: The Social and Political Construction of Women's Reproductive Choices

The social and political construction of female reality is a basic tenet of modern feminism. The feminist saying, "the personal is political," reveals that women's choices have not only been socially but politically orchestrated as well. When men and women act in certain ways, they are more than mere products of their socialization. Social conditioning theories often lack a political framework. Male domination and female subordination are bound up with power. There are positive advantages in status, ego, and authority for men in the ways, for example, they exercise their sexuality. The male power modes of sexuality construct women's sexual and reproductive lives to conform to male dictates.

When radical feminists stress how women's reproductive choices are influenced by the social and political system and how women are channeled into having children at any cost to themselves, we are reproached for portraying women as victims. These reproaches have come mainly from feminist liberals but, increasingly, they are being echoed by liberal men. In the Baby M case, Gary Skoloff, the lawyer for Bill Stern, summed up his court argument by stating, "If you prevent women from becoming surrogate mothers . . . you are saying that they do not have the ability to make their own decisions. . . . It's being unfairly paternalistic and it's an insult to the female population of this nation."[34] Skoloff probably learned this lingo from liberal lawyer Lori Andrews, who wrote, "Great care needs to be taken not to portray women as incapable of responsible decisions."[35]

Choice occurs in the context of a society where, to put it mildly, there are fundamental differences of power between men and women. Yet feminists who oppose technological and contractual reproduction are vilified for supposedly claiming that "infertile women and, by implication, all women [are] incapable of rationally grounded and authentic choice."[36] Little is said about why women are willing to submit their bodies to the most invasive and harmful medical interventions—for example, because their lives are devalued without children, because of husband/family pressure, because there has been little research and few resources devoted to infertility, and because women are channeled into abusive technologies at any cost to themselves. There is the presumption that if women choose to treat their bodies in this way—as reproductive experiments, vehicles, or objects for another's use—this is not problematic. This argument *is* problematic, however, because it minimizes the social and political contexts in which women's choices are made. Even the New Jersey Supreme Court decision, *In the Matter of Baby M*, recognized that although many women make a choice to enter surrogate arrangements and many others do not perceive surrogacy as exploitative, this "does not diminish its potential for devaluation to other women."[37]

In addition to surrogacy and the new reproductive technologies, sexual and reproductive liberals have also claimed that women freely choose to enter pornography. This idea of pornography as a woman's unadulterated choice appeared most prominently in a document called the FACT (Feminist Anti-Censorship Taskforce) Brief. FACT organized for the sole purpose of defeating the Dworkin-MacKinnon feminist antipornography ordinance that makes pornography legally actionable as a violation of women's civil rights. Throughout the FACT Brief, the rhetoric of false victimization prevails. "The ordinance . . . reinforces sexist images of women as incapable of consent. . . . In effect, the ordinance creates a strong presumption that women who participate in the creation of sexually explicit material [FACT's euphemism for pornography] are coerced."[38] The FACT Brief went so far as to say that women have been stereotyped as victims by the statutory rape laws.

Radical feminists stress how male supremacy channels women into pornography and surrogacy as well as into other reproductive procedures, while liberals charge that radical feminists make women into victims. There is a mechanism of denial operating in these accusations. In saying that women are not victims of male dominance, the liberal critics absolve themselves of responsibility for the victims. They obscure the necessity to create social and political change for those who are victims and they disidentify with their own victimization.

The kind of choice that feminist critics of technological and contractual reproduction would defend is substantive, not a so-called woman's choice growing out of a context of powerlessness. Instead, the more substantive question is, Do such so-called choices as surrogacy foster the empowerment of women as a group and create a better world for women? What kind of choices do women have when subordination, poverty, and degrading work are the options available to many? The point is not to deny that women are capable of choosing within contexts of powerlessness, but to question how much real value, worth, and power these so-called choices have.

Women make choices about what they judge to be in their own self-interest or survival, often in a desperate attempt to find safety or security, and often to give meaning to their existence. Andrea Dworkin, in

Right-Wing Women, demonstrates that politically conservative as well as feminist women are aware of the ways in which women are subordinated to male dictates, yet the former make different choices than feminists do. They choose what they perceive to be in their own best interests. Like most women, they make survival choices in a context of restricted options. So are we then to anoint their choices merely because they freely choose? In a similar way, *because* some women choose to enter surrogate contracts or submit themselves to the bodily invasions of multiple IVF treatments does not validate those choices.

In one way, this discussion of the social and political construction of women's choices demonstrates the old philosophical debate between freedom and necessity. Necessity is imposed through the social forces that dictate the conditions of women's lives, conditions that women do not create. That women do not often create the social conditions within which they act does not abrogate their capacity to choose, but it does call for a more complex assessment of what we call women's choices, bidding us to focus less on choice and more on its constraints. What are the organized forces shaping women's choice of surrogacy and other reproductive techniques? For starters, the whole social context of sexual subordination in which women live their lives and which results, for many, in economic poverty, dead-ended jobs, and low self-esteem. In surrogate agencies, there is a conjunction of male medical, corporate, and legal interests promoting the reproductive management of women. The media put on a promotional show, as well.

This is not to say that women who sign surrogate contracts are *simply* passive victims. Women's victimization can be acknowledged without labeling women passive. *Passive* and *victim* do not necessarily go together. Jews were victims of the Nazis, but they were not passive, nor did the reality of victimization define the totality of their existence. Blacks were victims of slavery, yet no thoughtful commentator would ever portray slaves as passive. It seems obvious that women can be victims of pornography and technological reproduction without depriving women of some ability to act under oppressive conditions, else how could any woman extract herself from these conditions, as many have?

Feminists can move beyond a one-dimensional focus on women's oppression without relinquishing the critique of women's oppression. This is the most serious failure of sexual and reproductive liberalism—

the relinquishing of the critique of the oppression of women. The end result of this abdication is that while lip service may be paid in minimal ways to the "possible" abuses of surrogacy and the new reproductive technologies, the present ways in which women do move beyond sexual and reproductive violence are never validated. For example, the sexual and reproductive liberal literature does not mention the exsurrogates and the expornography models who have organized to fight against surrogacy and pornography instead of promoting these as economic options for women. Many women who have been victims of pornography and surrogacy have become the systems' most powerful critics, but we are, instead, urged to examine the ways in which these systems of pornography and surrogacy, for example, are useful to women.

Finally, it seems obvious that one can recognize women's victimization by these institutions without shoring up the institutions themselves. When the sexual and reproductive liberals affirm that women are agents in a "culture" of pornography and technological reproduction, they sideline the agency of the institutions, thereby letting them off the hook. Why find evidence of women's agency *within* institutions of women's oppression and then use that agency to bolster these very systems? Why not locate women's agency in resistance to these institutions—for example, the agency of women who have courageously testified about their abuse in pornography and surrogacy, risking exposure and ridicule and often getting it; the exsurrogates who have fought for themselves and their children in court against the far greater advantages of the sperm source. Why locate women's agency primarily within the "culture" of male supremacy? And why shift attention from an analysis and activism aimed at destroying these systems to a justification of them? By romanticizing the victimization of women as liberating, sexual and reproductive liberalism leaves women in these systems at the mercy of them.

Sexual and reproductive liberalism has produced a new idealization of women's oppression; it defends the institution of surrogacy as providing the means for women's economic survival and the institution of pornography as freeing the expression of a repressed outlaw female sexuality.[39] This idealization makes women's subordination and abuse honorable, much in the tradition of the nineteenth-century view of ennobling women's domestic confinement and "conservation of energy." If oppression produces sexually or reproductively "free" women, it is a grand case for more oppression—not for ending the sexual and repro-ductive subordination of women.

When pornography and surrogacy are idealized as choices, this defines a new range of conformity for women. Choice is not the same as self-determination. Choice can be conformity if women have little abil-ity to determine the conditions of consent. A woman may consent to use the pill or the IUD as a contraceptive, after having the risks explained to her, but she has no sexual and reproductive self-determination if she cannot say no to intercourse with her male partner. A woman who signs a surrogate contract, agreeing to bear a child for a contracting couple, consents to the arrangement, but she has little self-determination if she cannot find sustaining and dignified work and resorts to surrogacy as a final economic resort. Feminists must go beyond choice and consent as a standard for women's freedom. Before consent, there must be self-determination so that consent does not simply amount to acquiescing to the available options.

When technological reproduction perpetuates the role of women as breeders or encourages women to have children at any cost, this is not reproductive self-determination. It is conformity to old social roles garbed in new technologies and the new language of individual rights and choice. Under the guise of fostering procreative liberty, these reproductive arrangements help mold women to traditional reproduc-tive roles. The fact that this compliance is ratified with the victim's con-sent only serves to emphasize how deeply conformity is entrenched and concealed in a gender-defined society.

Technological and contractual reproduction promotes the ideology that the problem of infertility *cannot* be confronted on an autonomous level but needs the intervention of medical and technical specialists to remedy the lack of biological children. Other options—an existence without children, an informed adoption—are not promoted as favorable alternatives. And thus women are left with the hollow rhetoric of choice—in reality, no choice at all.

Coercion and Complicity

Some critics of technological reproduction use the language of coercion to explain why women enter IVF programs or consent to surrogate con-tracts. Their attempt to show how choices are constrained for women under present social conditions is worthwhile, yet I do not find the language of coercion in the context of reproductive procedures particularly helpful. The degree and conditions of constraints on women are very different in the context of technological reproduction than, for example, in the context of pornography and prostitution. Most women in these latter systems have an extreme history of coercion, including rape, battery, incest, and child sexual abuse. Women are coerced into pornography and prostitution by pimps, lovers, husbands, fathers, as well as others:

> Pimps roam bus stations to entrap young girls who left incestuous homes thinking nothing could be worse. Pornographers advertise for lingerie or art or acting models they then bind, assault, and photograph, demanding a smile as the price for sparing their life. Men roam the highways with penises and cameras in hand, raping women with both at once. Husbands force their wives to pose as part of coerced sex, often enforced by threats to the lives of their children. Women are abducted by pimps from shopping centers and streets at random, sometimes never to return. Young women are tricked or pressured into posing for boyfriends and told that the pictures are just "for us," only to find themselves in this month's *Hustler*.[40]

The political and social construction of women's options in systems of reproduction, however, is not the same degree of coercion to which women are subjected in systems of sexual subordination, such as pornography and prostitution. Surrogacy comes closest in the instances where women have been deceived about their role or threatened after they have signed the contract. Women who undergo IVF procedures, however, are not coerced in this sense of extreme exploitation. In fact, women in IVF are complicitous to a certain extent that, nonetheless, does not deny the reality of the constraints or the ways in which women's choices are managed by the medical establishment.

Understanding women's complicity can help us to discern the different ways in which women come to accept what men want us to accept. This is neither to blame women, as the sexual and reproductive liberals do, nor to accept the institutions of women's reproductive oppression—the IVF mills and the systems of surrogacy—because women in these contexts are not outrightly coerced in the extreme. It is to say that pressure exists in many ways, not only at the level of coercion. It is also to make distinctions, reasserting the difference between social determinism and social constructionism. To affirm that women's choices and consent can be constructed, influenced, and pressured is not the same as to claim that women's choices are ruled by these social and political conditions. That reproductive arrangements are shaped by male power contextualizes but does not determine women's participation in these arrangements.

On the other hand, the language of coercion in the context of technological reproduction says too little about the complexity of consent. As one woman doctor who had undergone infertility treatments explained, "Looking back over the events . . . I by no means consider myself a passive victim, but know that I *actively* subjected myself to this violation of my body."[41] She then recounts a course of "violently enforced action" to conceive a child without letting her own subjectivity and agency off the hook. In retrospect, she realizes her own complicity in these reproductive manipulations.

Although women may participate in medical violations of their own bodies, many change and become resisters. The explanation of coercion flattens out the truth that women do act under conditions of oppression, but that their actions are qualified in significant ways. If surrogacy and IVF are violations of human dignity and bodily integrity, the violations occur whether they happen personally or to others. By participating in the exploitation of the self, one contributes to the exploitation of others. When women recognize their own complicity in their own oppression, often this recognition is a consciousness-raising event. For many, it enables them to get out from under the oppression.

Critiquing a theory of history that sees the self only as a product of socially constructed interactions with others and events, sociologist Kathleen Barry states, "Selves [in these theories] are not more than their material and social realities. . . . With that, the future is rejected for women if they cannot project beyond the present and, therefore, beyond domination." Barry contends that "women usually know more about domination than they speak . . . ," since women's subordination has been personalized and made private and intimate. The consciousness of oppression, spoken or not, creates a historical dynamism; theories about the social construction of women's choices, no matter how radical they are, cannot essentialize a woman's self, making social conditions determinative of her total reality. "With an interactive concept of the self in praxis, we can begin to study the social construction of women in a historical context and, thereby, discover that which enables and that which prevents any woman from becoming a 'woman unto herself.'"[42]

Understanding the complexity of women's consent involves exposing the conditions of oppression that constrain women and their choices as well as attending to the ways in which women act and change—for good or for ill—as they gain or deny awareness and historical consciousness of what has been done to them. In some circumstances, it involves admitting women's complicity in our own oppression. Complicity has been women's stake in the system.

Although the sexual and reproductive liberals lay claim to a nuanced view of women's oppression, they treat the social and political construction of women's consent as unproblematic. There is a constant pretension to complexity in their work, but it is as if, paying lip service to the rhetoric of complexity, they do not understand the reality of complexity in women's lives. Relying on a liberal theory of choice, they blame women and do not recognize the constraints on women's choices. Instead of looking at the complexity of women's agency under the conditions of oppression, they fault women for "getting themselves into these situations" or valorize the situations as liberating to women in ways "unintended by the patriarchs." They do not valorize women who resist, who bring suit against the surrogate brokers, who testify about their abuse in pornography, and who work for legislation to prosecute surrogate brokers, pimps, and pornographers. They simplify complexity.

The sexual and reproductive liberals also *reduce complexity to relativism*. The fact that many women make different choices under conditions of oppression leads the liberals to an ethical and political relativism that claims it is impossible to make judgments about women's participation in prostitution and reproductive technologies and thus about the systems themselves. There is no right or wrong in their view, just simple difference. Surrogacy is neither good nor bad for women, they say. Different women make different choices.

Different women do make different choices, and this suggests that we live in a world of ethical and political complexity rather than of moral relativity. Complexity demands that we search for moral and political answers to the various facets of reproductive trafficking instead of ignoring the search or reducing it to "everything is relative." Complexity demands moral discernment and the political courage to make judgments about what is oppressive or beneficial to women and then to act on these judgments.

CHAPTER 4

The Marketing of the
New Reproductive Technologies:
Medicine, the Media, and
the Idea of Progress

All the reproductive technologies and contracts discussed thus far are portrayed as technological breakthroughs that provide new choices for women. In the West, images of progress pervade their representation in the print and electronic media, and in the name of progress many new reproductive procedures have become covered under some health insurance plans.

Progress, however, is elusive. Philosophers write about it as an idea, yet I think progress is most fully captured by the theological vision of eschatology. Within Christian theology, eschatology is what is hoped for, what fulfills the future, or the goal of history realized in the Kingdom of God, eternal life, and the second coming of Jesus. One way to examine reproductive technologies is to study how they often function as eschatological statements—more promise than performance. This is especially evident in the language, images, and themes used to convey the media's representation of the new reproductive technologies. It is more patent in the past histories of promising drugs and technologies that turned perilous or were ultimately ineffective.

Images of the New Reproductive Technologies

Reigning themes and repetitive images in newspaper and magazine articles shape public consumption of the new reproductive technologies. Dorothy Nelkin, in her work *Selling Science: How the Press Covers Science and Technology,* points out that science journalists broker technological issues for their readers and help mold public consciousness about science and technology. Reporters do not act alone, however, but in turn scientists help shape their reporting.[1] In an age of competitive research funding and the race for public support, fame, and favorable press coverage, scientists have set up vast public information networks through their respective institutions that have been successful in marketing technology to the public through the media.

It is not that all science journalists are unreliable or that important knowledge cannot be gleaned from newspaper and magazine articles. In fact, I have culled from many print and electronic sources crucial and ground-breaking articles that have supported information gathered from both personal contacts and professional data. And some media sources are more reliable than academic and professional journals, which seldom confront critical issues in a direct way but instead accommodate their analysis to the prevailing point of view in the field, lack nerve, and are often out-of-date. Rather, in this chapter I point out how science and medical reporting, *as a genre,* has been enormously dependent on its scientific and medical sources, with the result that much of this reporting has been skewed in a scientifically self-interested direction. Because of the complexity of scientific and medical knowledge, but also because of the immense public relations industry set up to channel science and medical news to reporters and to the public, science and medical journalism has perhaps been more indebted to the hand that feeds it than other kinds of journalism.

Nelkin characterizes the relationship between scientists and the media as a *promotional model.* Science journalism in the United States and in many other Western countries generally promotes the great promise of technological breakthroughs. Many articles convey the message that technology is instrumental in constructing a better world. Social critics Noam Chomsky and Edward Herman in their analysis of the overall media go further and develop a *propaganda model.* They refer to the symbiotic relationship between the media and powerful sources of information as "shaping the supply of experts."[2] The media uses those who have vested interests in the technologies as experts who elaborate and define the issues for the public.

The promotional/propaganda message of the media is often polarized: "We read of either promising application or perilous effects, of triumphant progress or tragic risks. . . . The long-term political and social consequences of technological choices are seldom explored."[3] And the message of peril is usually not heard until after the fact.

Press coverage of new reproductive technologies initially uses a language of promise. In some articles, risk is warned about, but mostly in a futuristic or abstract sense with rare reference to the historical context of past technologies gone wrong. Reproductive and genetic engineering news is often covered as a series of dramatic events with the stress on technological miracle, magic, and mystique. Today, reproductive and genetic engineering has become a national symbol of progress, comparable to the space program of the 1960s and '70s.

For example, Keith Schneider, who has often written science pieces for the *New York Times,* wrote an article, "Repro Madness," for the U.S. *New Age Journal.* In spite of the title, which might indicate a critical perspective, the bulk of the six-page article is a promotional brief for the techniques, especially those provided by the Comprehensive Fertility Institute directed by lawyer Bill Handel in Los Angeles. The institute is mainly a surrogate brokerage agency, selling the reproductive services of women to people who can pay. Although the article gives the appearance of a balanced presentation by quoting two critics of the technologies, their words are restricted to two short paragraphs.

Metaphors and discourse of progress pervade Schneider's article. New reproductive technologies constitute a "reproductive revolution." Humanity is propelled to the "edges of an altogether new frontier." Schneider even invokes religious metaphors, calling the developments godlike. This is a "pivotal period in which ordinary men and women will mimic God, actually designing sons and daughters in their own images."[4]

Exaggerated claims abound. It is as if the technological Kingdom of God is truly at hand. The fertility enterprises promoted in Schneider's article will soon be capable of pinpointing many genetic "defects." After that, parents will not only be able to correct chromosomal abnormalities but also choose from a list of "hereditary options" such as blue eyes, blond hair, high intelligence, physical strength, and even delayed aging. "An entire generation of supersmart, superstrong babies is a distinct possibility." And futuristic alternatives hold promise of artificial wombs in which "customized embryos" can grow to term. "No fuss. Satisfaction guaranteed."[5] The reproductive supermarket has arrived.

There is much homogeneity in popular magazine claims for new reproductive technologies, even from one industrialized country to another. Although the style and details may differ in these articles, most of them focus on the same assertions, pursue the same sources of information, and review the technologies in similar ways. In an article on embryo research written in *Vogue Australia*, we see a familiar pattern of hyperbole, enthusiasm, and list of futuristic possibilities as in the U.S. *New Age Journal*. Research on embryos "could lead" to a better understanding of miscarriage and infertility, the development of new contraceptives, and the treatment of disorders in infants. In addition, it may also help treat cancer and heart disease. "In time" embryo research could "wipe out" disabilities such as Down's syndrome, cystic fibrosis, hemophilia, and sickle-cell anemia. "In theory" children would no longer be born with inherited physical or mental handicaps.[6] "In theory," the shopping list is endless. And the story sells, so the media have little motivation to change.

While scientific rationality is supposedly the basis of medical journal articles, scientific romanticism pervades the popular press. Metaphors of "conquests" for all sorts of diseases, of reproductive technologies on the "frontier" of life, and of "miracle" babies celebrate unlimited possibilities of progress. Yet much of this progress is postponed to future development, future research, and future funding. Each new technology *promises* a transformation of existence.

The romanticized language of popular articles such as the *New Age Journal* and *Vogue Australia* is often routinized in mainstream newspaper articles that report on the success rates of, for example, in vitro fertilization. Although the 1985 Corea and Ince investigation documented widespread misrepresentation of success rates by IVF centers (see chapter 1), newspapers continued to report exaggerated figures after this survey had been published and after the U.S. Office of

Technology Assessment had confirmed these findings in 1988. Only in 1989 were conservative success rates acknowledged in the press. But these studies appear not to have affected any change in the public's attitude after having been so inundated with IVF progress stories.

Other newspaper accounts focus on the bigger and better claims for reproductive technologies. In May 1984 Australian newspapers carried lead articles entitled, "In-vitro Babies Better Adjusted" (*Canberra Times*); "Babies: They're Better from Glass" (*Sydney Morning Herald*); and "Test-tube Babies Are Smarter and Stronger"(*The Australian*). Four years later, in 1988, Carl Wood, one of Australia's leading IVF "pioneers," described artificial conception as "superior to natural conception" in attacking the Victorian government's control of the technology. Later in 1988 Wood contended that not only were the babies superior, but infertile couples are better equipped for the task of parenting because they are "quite different to the fly-by-night parents of naturally-conceived children who succeed with little thought and brief pleasure."[7]

As so often happens with science journalism, the media pendulum swings from eschatological endorsement to disillusionment. One year after the original newspaper accounts in 1984 that promoted the "superior babies" story, headlines in the Australian press shifted to: "IVF Babies Four Times More Likely to Die at Birth." These headlines were prompted by an Australian perinatal study (see chapter 1) documenting many problems with IVF babies.[8] Later, the coverage shifted back to endorsement as usual. In 1989, one year after Carl Wood's claim about the superiority of IVF babies, articles became more critical due to the initiative of feminist groups such as FINRRAGE, Australia. The media coverage of Wood's hyperbolic claims for IVF babies was designed to raise public expectation and cultivate public support. These claims were met with unqualified press optimism until the national perinatal study and the FINRRAGE criticism became public. Then the press shifted to the opposite standpoint, using language such as "cruel illusion" or "naive exaggeration" to speak of technologies gone wrong without acknowledging that the press had been party to the exaggerations and illusion. Usually, it is only after years of media endorsement and promotion that dissident studies and groups are given a hearing.

Chomsky and Herman have documented that only certain victims of political atrocities received widespread U.S. media coverage during the 1980s. For example, in examining the differences in quantity and tone of articles, number of front-page articles, and actual column inches given to what they call "worthy" (Eastern European) versus "unworthy" (Latin American) victims, Chomsky and Herman document the ways in which articles focused on Eastern European while downplaying Latin American atrocities. No quantitative study has been conducted that specifies the difference in coverage given to supporters and critics of technological and contractual reproduction. In the accounts that I examined, however, critical reporting on new reproductive procedures was vastly underrepresented and understated.

By diminishing the objections and the critical viewpoints, much media coverage effectively amounts to promotional news and censorship of dissenting viewpoints.[9] The coverage cocreates the reality.

Even when risks and criticisms are published, the power of technology's promise continues to linger. Doubt must translate into almost absolute peril before a technology loses its promise. In the wake of reported studies on the risks and dangers of IVF—to babies, not to women—Americans read in the 1990 *U.S. News and World Report* Health Almanac, entitled "Your A-Z Guide to Health":

> Researchers at Eastern Virginia Medical School in Norfolk, Va., have quelled fears that test-tube babies would not develop normally. In a study comparing 93 children ages 1 to 2½ with 83 conceived in vitro, they found no significant differences in physical or mental development. In fact, the test-tube kids generally had slightly higher IQ scores.[10]

What then are we to conclude? IVF babies are better in the United States than in Australia? Our clinics make babies better than they do? Popular press articles provide the public with high or low drama but with few ways to interpret the findings. Risk, unlike promise, is ignored or downplayed.

Many articles in U.S. newspapers use language akin to the promotional advertising of the infertility businesses. For example, a *Los Angeles Times* article was headlined "Surrogate Mother Extols 'Joy of Life' in Novel Experience." This article featured a "happy surrogate mother" who described the baby she had conceived and delivered for clients as "the son of a friend of our family, but one who I'm more interested in. . . ."[11] The "happy surrogate," a mainstay of the surrogate industry's advertising, has also become a regular feature of many newspaper articles intended to offset the bad publicity engendered by the 1987–88 Baby M legal battles. The promotional message of the *Los Angeles Times* article was achieved by exclusively featuring the director of the infertility operation, Bill Handel, and his employees. Another article from the *Los Angeles Herald Examiner* stated quite bluntly in its subtitle, "Unlike Baby M, Most Cases End Happily." This article spent its print telling the reader that although the Baby M tale is a sad one, it "appears to misrepresent the typical surrogate birthing experience." The final line concluded, "No matter how many times there's a birth, . . . it always is a miracle."[12]

Personal accounts of women who work as so-called surrogate mothers or stories of the rare infertile couples who obtained babies through the IVF process with smiling infant on lap serve as potent biographical and pictorial accounts of technological progress. Most often missing from these accounts are the numbers of dissatisfied customers and unhappy women who have worked as surrogates for infertility enterprises. Although the media feature accounts of exsurrogates such as Patty Foster, Alejandra Muñoz, Kathleen King, and Anna Johnson, as well as others who ultimately challenge this happy picture of surrogacy, their testimonies have no cumulative weight. Usually they are treated as isolated accounts in discrete and local media and seldom are included, beyond a fleeting reference, in national full-length, prominently placed feature articles on technological and contractual reproduction.

Also missing from the media coverage is a long historical view that provides a retrospective on the past history of reproductive drugs and techniques. It is an unfortunate lesson learned from this history that failure is often recognized after the fact of damage—damage that indeed had been evident, but not publicized, all along. It is instructive to look back on the history of much eschatological technology, reproductive as well as otherwise, once touted as miraculous, but often saving no one.

Memory Versus Forgetfulness: From Miracle to Mess

The artificial heart is one fairly recent case of unrealized medical eschatology. A decade ago, its coming was greeted with the prophecy that the technological Kingdom of God was at hand. The heart would replace cardiac surgery. The heart would prevent death. And the classic promise—the benefits (future) outweigh the risks (present). No matter that the first recipient died. That only served to canonize him and the heart. The publicity surrounding Barney Clark, the first martyr to the artificial heart, enhanced the expectations surrounding this technology because he had died "so that others might live." With more money, more research, and (nobody said this) more heroic victims, the heart's promise would be realized.

In January 1990 the U.S. government announced to the heart's maker, Symbion, Inc., that the promise of the artificial heart had *not* been fulfilled. The risks to patients were outweighing the benefits. Almost a decade and 250 million research dollars later, there are no more prophetic statements about the artificial heart. Many hearts have been recalled, and the National Institutes of Health no longer support it with grants. The euphoria has died off and the heart no longer beats with government assistance.

More recently, in 1992, there was the culmination of the breast implant debacle. In the 1970s, 350,000 women underwent silicone breast reconstructive surgery after breast cancer and, in the same period, more than one million women had them implanted to increase the size of their breasts.[13] During this same decade, serious problems were reported with their use: leaking implants, migration of the silicone, infections, autoimmune disorders, painful scar tissue, and loss of nerve sensation in the breasts. Against the tide of overwhelming evidence that silicone breast implants were dangerous to women's health, the well-financed plastic surgery industry and Dow Corning, the major manufacturer of the silicone implants, continued to defend their widespread use. Even after a decade of FDA hearings that documented the risks and dangers of the implants to women, the American Society of Plastic and Reconstructive Surgeons initiated a four million dollar lobbying campaign in 1991 to keep the implants on the market.[14]

By the end of 1991, however, the FDA had obtained internal documents from Dow Corning, dating back to 1975, describing concerns and criticisms expressed by Dow's own scientists about the safety of the breast implants. The FDA found that other company scientists had misrepresented a key animal study in which dogs given implants had actually died when, in a medical journal article, the dogs were reported to be in normal health. Dow Corning had also failed to conduct critical safety tests, had cut corners, and had concealed risks on all levels. Finally, in April 1992 the FDA banned most silicone breast implants, although they can still be used to reconstruct the breasts of women after breast cancer surgery and in what are called "controlled clinical experiments."[15]

Although the silicone breast implant business depended on those women whose lives had been ravaged by breast cancer, only to be ravaged again by silicone breast insertion, the bulk of the profits were built on the bodies of the 80 percent of women without breast cancer who used them for breast augmentation. According to the American Society of Plastic and Reconstructive Surgeons, small breasts are not only "deformities" but "*a disease* which in most patients results in feelings of inadequacy."[16] This attitude graphically represents the tendency of many researchers and physicians to build their medical practice on the sexual objectification and mutilation of women's bodies.

In the months after the end of World War II, Japanese doctors and cosmetologists reportedly began injecting silicone into the breasts of prostitutes.[17] It seems that the occupying American GIs took no pleasure in small-breasted Japanese women, so industrial-strength silicone coolant was injected directly into their breasts.[18] The next group of women whose breasts were mauled were an estimated 50,000 topless dancers, waitresses, and entertainers in Nevada, made famous by the bust of Carol Doda, who was transformed into an "icon of silicone" when her breast size went from 34B to 44D.

The breast implant saga is fresh in our memories, but a host of other failed drugs and technologies were used on women in the past. The enchantment with new reproductive technologies is, in part, a contest of memory versus forgetfulness—forgetfulness of past failures versus a memory of promise. Today's promise is too often tomorrow's peril. Nowhere have these technological and chemical perils loomed larger than in reproductive medicine and in technologies that have been developed for women.

There was the promise of diethylstilbestrol (DES), a drug initially given to pregnant women to prevent miscarriage. The tragic history of this drug is well known because it caused cancer and infertility in many DES daughters. Thalidomide was even more graphic in its consequences. Given as a sedative during pregnancy to thousands of

European women, it led to the death and disfigurement of their children. Contraceptives like the Dalkon Shield, the pill, and Depo-Provera have all been the subject of public debate in the United States. Some, like the Dalkon Shield, have been proven to the satisfaction of the so-called experts to be more recognizably dangerous than the pill. This enlightenment often occurs when the victims of these technologies and drugs pursue litigation. Studies continue to find pill links with cancer, only to be challenged by other studies. This has been the contradictory professional certification of the pill since the 1960s.

Depo-Provera, another promising drug, was initially banned as a contraceptive until 1992 when the FDA approved it. During the time of its ban in the United States, it was exported to Third World women. When reproductive progress is countermanded in the First World, we often export our so-called progress to the supposedly unprogressive Third World. Moreover, as the National Black Women's Health Project has revealed, although Depo-Provera was not licensed for contraceptive use in the United States prior to 1992, many African American women regularly received the drug from their doctors.[19] In 1987 the U.S. Indian Health Service was also continuing to prescribe Depo-Provera as a contraceptive for Native American women.[20] When officially banned, Depo-Provera remained a contraceptive given to Third World women in the so-called First World.

There is more. Once touted as necessary to 25 percent of the birthing women in the United States, half of the one million cesarian deliveries are today recognized as unnecessary.[21] The diagnostic value of the electronic fetal monitor is now debated.[22] And in a major shift of policy, a U.S. Public Health Service panel of experts has recently recommended *less* prenatal care for most healthy pregnant women. It acknowledges that many procedures and tests performed on healthy pregnant women, such as routine screening for protein in the urine at every prenatal visit, multiple pap tests, and more than one pelvic examination, are expensive, time consuming, and provide no real benefit.[23]

As a study in eschatological journalism, the case of estrogen replacement therapy bears closer examination. Coverage of estrogen replacement therapy (now called hormonal replacement therapy) began in 1963. The journalistic hype in this case relied on the progressive image of estrogen replacement therapy (ERT) as a "cure for growing old." Typical headlines were: "Women Forever Young" and "Preventing Menopause." An Associated Press (AP) article quoted as fact the statement of a scientist asserting that "there is no reason why they [women] should grow old."[24] This article and others portrayed doctors who were reluctant to prescribe estrogen to decrease the effects of menopause and aging as archaic. The news media emphasized estrogen's progressive role in keeping women young.

This message was very popular with female readers, but it was also a message calculated to make headlines. The major experts promoting ERT and making their materials available to the news media were two doctors who stood to gain much from the coverage. Author of the well-known book *Feminine Forever*, Dr. Robert Wilson was a gynecologist whose research on estrogen was funded by drug firms.[25] In fact, he directed a foundation whose sole mission was to publish and distribute reports and recommendations about specific products, among them ERT. He and other scientists minimized the links between estrogens and cancer that were increasingly becoming known. As a result of their massive public relations efforts in which they mailed advocacy materials to newspapers, but especially to women's magazines throughout the country, many promotional articles appeared. The slogan became: "Femininity need not fade at fifty."

Dr. Robert A. Kistner, a professor of gynecology at the Harvard Medical School, also stood to benefit. A regular consultant to drug companies, he wrote many popular articles on ERT that appeared in women's magazines.[26] Even after the U.S. Food and Drug Administration (FDA) had issued warnings about the relationship between ERT and endometrial cancer in 1969, he publicly criticized the warnings and the studies they were based on.

Popular articles continued to promote ERT after the much-publicized U.S. congressional hearings in 1970 that brought more public attention to the negative effects of estrogen drugs. "The press responded, conveying the message that using estrogen for birth control could be harmful for health."[27] But using estrogen for menopause continued to be recommended for "extra years of vitality," and the cancer worries were called a "needless fear."[28] Even when a 1975 article in the *New England Journal of Medicine* definitively linked ERT to increased risk of endometrial cancer and was widely summarized in the popular mainstream press, many doctors said they would still prescribe ERT.[29]

In 1976, Ayerst Laboratories, the manufacturer of estrogen drugs, hired the public relations company of Hill and Knowlton to counteract the unfavorable publicity. Hill and Knowlton recommended that Ayerst contact science editors of major newspapers, avoid any direct promotion of the use of estrogens, and instead focus on menopause using the technique of "discrete reference" to its estrogen therapy.[30] In other words, they encouraged press coverage that sidestepped questions about the ill effects of estrogen.

Estrogen replacement therapy was resurrected in the 1980s as "hormonal replacement therapy" (HRT), a new name and supposedly a new drug. By mixing estrogen with progestin, the drug companies hoped to circumvent earlier warnings about ERT. Now the press cited problems with estrogen taken *alone* but promoted the new mix of estrogen and progestin as a different and less risky treatment. "But many of the questions regarding safety are still unanswered, and the proponents of the combined therapy fail to recognize the absurdity of using one synthetic hormone, progesterone, to combat the ill-effects of another synthetic hormone, estrogen."[31]

Whereas the media had earlier promoted ERT as reversing the effects of aging, it now focused on HRT's role in preventing osteoporosis. Ayerst again conducted a public relations campaign through major U.S. women's magazines such as *Redbook* and *Women's Day* trumpeting the use of its drug, Premarin, for the debilitating disease of osteoporosis. For women in the 1960s and '70s, the debilitating disease was aging; in the '80s, it was osteoporosis.

The active role of the pharmaceutical industry and its mediation in the press have been crucial in constructing ruinous female pathologies for which drugs become the major answer. The two go together—the creation of the debilitating disease and then the arresting drug. Promoters of HRT view menopause itself as the pathology, a deficiency disease that afflicts all women. However, the disease and the drug are modified depending on time, place, and the pendulum swing of the media's representation from progress to peril.

Once more, after an initial outburst of favorable HRT coverage in the early 1980s, the press began to chronicle studies of more unfavorable developments. In 1989 the *Washington Post,* repeating articles that had appeared in other major mainstream media, reported, "Hormone Use in Menopause Tied to Cancer."[32] The full study, which had been published in the *New England Journal of Medicine*, found that "combination therapy" may increase the results of developing breast cancer. Other reports maintained that while estrogen might increase a woman's chances of developing breast cancer, it helped to ward off heart disease. Depending on how the press framed the headlines about a 1991 study, one read either that "Estrogen After Menopause Cuts Heart Attack Risk, Study Finds,"[33] or that "Doubt Remains About Estrogen for Menopause."

Coverage of estrogen and, later, hormonal replacement therapy is only one instance of many in which science reporters have jumped on the bandwagon of female reproductive progress, only later to uncover the perils of this progress. Many other examples could be cited of the media's promotion of reproductive drugs and technologies that have gone down in history as major technological and media mistakes. Given the public relations campaigns of the medical and technological promoters and their success in "shaping the supply of experts," this progressive coverage is not surprising.

What is to be learned from this past history of so-called progress? First, scientists and the media use the same eschatological language today to sell the wonders of reproductive technologies, and a vulnerable infertile population is willing to try anything that offers a ray of hope and that is touted as innovation. In the debate over embryo research in England, a group called Progress claimed that embryo research was necessary to cure and prevent infertility, to prevent miscarriage, to improve contraception, and to conquer genetic disease. An embryologist, writing in the *New Scientist*, was prompted to observe, "Is this really the case? If we look behind the rhetoric it is clear that human embryologists are somewhat confused about what they intend to do next with the limited amount of experimental material available to them."[34]

Second, medical history is filled with examples of past miracle technologies that later proved disillusioning, if not outright dangerous. Yet, in responding to the history of estrogen replacement therapy, as well as to other technological and drug debacles, defenders of progress may be tempted to dismiss these examples as anecdotal or as exceptions to the progressive history of modern medicine. Unfortunately, they are as much the rule as they are the exception. Sociologist Diana Dutton has pointed out that it is possible to evaluate medical innovations beyond pointing to the individual examples of drugs and technologies that proved useless or dangerous. "According to a federally commissioned study, less than half of the drugs sold between 1938 and 1962 were effective for claimed therapeutic purposes. Similarly, careful evaluation of a broad range of modern medical and surgical innovations has shown that only half offered improvements over standard practice, even without considering the costs."[35] Much has also been written on technologies known to be ineffective that, once adopted, are discontinued not when they are disproven scientifically, but simply when they go out of fashion.[36]

This data and literature confirm what earlier critics of medical progress, such as René Dubos and Ivan Illich, have maintained. The most significant improvements have resulted from environmental and public health innovations and changes. As Dubos wrote, sanitation measures and changes in environmental conditions, not medical technical measures, accounted for most modern health improvements: "While modern science can boast of so many startling achievements in the health fields, its role has not been so unique and its effectiveness not so complete as is commonly claimed. In reality . . . the monstrous specter of infection had become but an enfeebled shadow of its former self by the time serums, vaccines, and drugs became available to combat microbes."[37]

In 1959, Dubos pointed out that an overall increase in life expectancy over the last hundred years was due to the decrease in infant mortality and control of childhood diseases that, in turn, resulted from better nutrition and sanitary practice rather than from the introduction of new drugs. He reminds us that very little progress has been made in the control of the adult killer diseases, such as cancer and heart ailments, since the work of the nineteenth-century public health and environmental reformers.

More recently, Thomas McKeown has shown that, for most disease, Western medicine's preoccupation with technological and therapeutic intervention is misguided and that more attention should be given to the effects of social and economic circumstances.[38] Yet for medical science and for most of the public, greater health and the conquest of disease mean more technology; "so deeply imbedded is the role of technology in our culture that the term 'innovation' is often used as if it were synonymous with technological innovation."[39] And the idea of progress is synonymous with technological advancement.

The charge of antitechnology has been crucial in discrediting opponents of the medical-technical fix. Science is intolerant of the views and values of those it dismisses as nonexperts, and critical perspectives are crowded out of the press.

Accusations of Antitechnology and the Reign of the Experts

Critics of technologies who warn about potential or existing damage and complications are generally termed Luddites (those who want to destroy technology), doomsayers, and antitechnological Cassandras (prophets who predict disaster but are not believed). The most tragic consequence of this name calling is that the defenders of reproductive technology are more concerned with criticizing the critics than they are with investigating the risks to women.

In his keynote address to the 1988 American Association for the Advancement of Science annual meeting, David Baltimore, who later became president of Rockefeller University (after having been implicated in a widely publicized case of scientific fraud, and eventually was forced to resign his presidency), said, "To me . . . the most powerful retrograde forces are outmoded ideas and concepts that clash with progressive thinking, attempting to suppress new knowledge and new concepts."[40] As the newly installed president of this scientific organization, Baltimore was taking up the cudgels to answer those critics of science who, in his opinion, are trying "to stop all DNA research . . . pitting laboratory investigators against those who see only hazards in new technology."[41] Along with the critics of DNA, Baltimore lumped in animal rightists, critics of biotechnology, critics of the human genome project and clone banks, and the creation science movement.

Baltimore sidestepped the real issues that underlie the critique of science: expertise versus elitism, entrenched professional priorities versus sociopolitical priorities, and lack of accountability versus the responsibility of scientists to the public. Journalists convey very little about the ethics and politics of science, the structure of scientific institutions, the priorities that guide technological decisions, and the ideologies of science in the making. The accusations of antitechnology portray critics as having a primitive mindset that stands in the way of progress.

For example, legislation regulating experiments on human embryos in Victoria was branded as "holding back research that could lead to important medical advances. . . ."[42] People who raise moral, social, and political objections to reproductive engineering are "rigid thinkers." Science writers quote self-serving sources like Dr. Richard Seed, proprietor of a fertility clinic in Chicago, who brands the critics:

> There's no controversy. . . . Forget this business about "that's illegal, immoral, and let's stop and think.". . . We should charge ahead and do it and forget about the moral minority who wants to live in the fifth century. . . . The greatest menace to progress is rigid thinking.[43]

Thus attentiveness to moral and social issues is characterized as rigid thinking rather than as an intelligence of values, priorities, and an emphasis on limits.

As the national debate rages over feasible and fair ways to limit expensive technology that benefits few people, the development of expensive and selective reproductive technologies continues at a reckless pace. In Europe, over 200,000 frozen embryos have been stockpiled in laboratories, with numbers heading into the millions. One IVF baby costs in excess of $50,000 U.S. dollars when the costs of increased hospitalization, increased obstetrical interventions at birth, and increased neonatal care are added in.[44] Israel, with a population of 4.4 million people, has an exorbitant number of eighteen IVF clinics.[45] Particularly in France and the United States, but in other countries as well, IVF enterprises, often offering other reproductive services such as surrogacy, continue to proliferate. A summary report of the World Health Organization defines IVF as *experimental*, taking the position that no new technology should become an accepted medical practice until it has undergone a thorough and careful scientific evaluation, which has not been the case with IVF. Instead, there has been an uncontrollable expansion of this technology.[46] The WHO report recommends that governments should limit the further proliferation of new IVF centers, determine the priority for infertility services within the context of all human services, limit the number of IVF treatment cycles for women, and restrict the indications for IVF.[47]

Reproductive technologies are running rampant by comparison with the limits and priorities being advocated in other areas of high technology delivery and practice. And these technologies are being framed in the contexts of rights and liberties—for example, the right to a child or the principle of procreative liberty—that have provided the ethical and legal grounding for reproductive technology entitlement in the United States. This entitlement is becoming more and more open-ended regardless of the economic cost and, more importantly, the cost to women's health and well-being.

We have, effectively, in the United States, a growing entitlement program based on fulfilling the desire of selective consumers for children, a desire that is always translated into need. Moreover, to say that we must meet all the desires of reproductive consumers, only some of whom are technically infertile, is to grant that which we would grant to no other medical interest group. For a society that must increasingly set technological and medical limits, it is the height of folly to create more programs and more entitlements to assure that everyone who desires a child should have one by any means possible.

Fear of being looked upon as antitechnology often induces skeptics to support reactionary technologies, finding use where there is abuse and benefit where there is risk. The antitechnology epithet is used as a control mechanism for marginalizing criticism. In the United States, being called antitechnology is almost like being called a Communist. It sets one at odds with all that is deemed good. The accusation helps mobilize the public against critics of particular technologies. Because the antitechnology idea is fuzzy, it can be used against anybody advocating even a thoughtful consideration of risks and benefits. Critics and concerned citizens are kept on the defensive by this label, under great pressure to pay homage to advances in technology. The not-so-subtle message of this antitechnology name calling is that sophisticated, progressive people are not opposed to anything technological. That's simplistic and does not account for the vast range of nuances that a more complex calculus of the issues would recognize. This sophistication, however, masks a passivity whereby the sophisticates actually capitulate to the technologies and philosophies of a progress that must march on at all costs, especially to female life and well-being.

The progress rhetoric bolstering technological reproduction often borders on technological determinism—equating the technical choice with the moral and social choice. The rhetoric of progress treats technological developments as mere scientific and technical considerations to be decided by the experts, not as moral and social judgments to be made by all those involved. The concerns of patients, involved citizens, and informed critics are systematically undervalued or ignored relative to the interests of the so-called experts. Feminist critics of reproductive technologies, for example, are often challenged on grounds of credentials. The assumption by the medical profession and the media is that feminists are biased outsiders and lack an expert professional point of view. Judged wanting in scientific competence, feminists are viewed as not entitled to speak on technological matters.

Meanwhile, certain technotwits are constantly quoted in the mainstream press. Science as an institution and the scientific experts are assumed to be neutral sources of authority. Scientists and scientific sympathizers act as gatekeepers who quash even their own internal dissenters while certifying quotable professional pundits to ensure an orthodox self-perpetuating view of the field.

Self-perpetuating experts and self-perpetuating views of science have political consequences. As Herman and Chomsky write, "The mass media are drawn into a symbiotic relationship with powerful sources of information by economic necessity and reciprocity of interest. The media need a steady, reliable flow of the raw material of news."[48] In turn, the scientists need the media and go to great lengths to get their own version of their particular technological story out to the public. The magnitude of the public information operations set up by hospitals, clinics, and research centers is designed for media access, but within the parameters dictated by the institutions. It overpowers any competition for media access from critics or dissenters, providing the media "with facilities in which to gather; they give journalists advance copies of speeches and forthcoming reports; they schedule press conferences at hours well-geared to news deadlines; they write press releases in usable language; and they carefully organize their press conferences and 'photo opportunity' sessions."[49] In addition, they even provide telephones and food. One reporter described these public information sessions to be "like covering a football game where they hand out statistics at the end of every quarter."[50] The emergence of media consultants—highly paid advice givers and strategists for scientific institutions and technical enterprises—has also significantly dampened any critical tendencies the press might have.

The dominance of scientific and scientific-sympathetic sources is offset, of course, by some critics who are highly respected and who lend a certain authority to dissident perspectives. George Wald, a Nobel Prize winner, is in this category. But the critics are in much shorter and much less visible supply than the official sources. Further, they are not as needed by the media because they are not the people who provide the media with the breaking news or raw data, that is, the latest miracle technologies or the technical explanations. By giving purveyors of technological reproduction a great deal of exposure, the press confers media expert status on them and makes them the preferred sources for further opinions and analysis.

The media do, however, have their favorite dissident pundits. Jeremy Rifkin has been widely quoted as a critical authority on biotechnology, genetic engineering, and reproductive procedures. Rifkin's Foundation on Economic Trends has made a science out of cultivating media contacts and presenting Rifkin himself as the major source to be contacted when a critical point of view is sought on these issues. Even when Rifkin forms coalitions, as has been his tactic in opposing, for example, the release of the ice-minus bacteria, he is headlined in the media as the spokesman for a group of environmentalists who filed suit, charging that NIH had not adequately evaluated the ecological consequences of the bacterial release.

Many newspaper editors also discourage any critical commentary by their reporters because of the threat and high cost of possible litigation. Reporters are discouraged from doing investigative journalism and instead engage in a highly orchestrated type of science reporting beholden to press releases, thus producing safe copy. Reporters ignore sources that argue contrary to the prevailing social and scientific values and also avoid writing about the complexity of the issues.

One stark example of an elaborate strategy of the experts speaking on behalf of their own interests was the publication of the American Fertility Society's report on the new reproductive technologies. Impressively entitled "Ethical Considerations of the New Reproductive Technologies," it was compared by journalists to the Warnock Report in Britain and the Waller Report in Australia, both produced by advisory ethics panels that were governmentally appointed. The American Fertility Society, in contrast, is no such independent group. It counts, among its membership of 10,000 physicians and scientists, a large number who develop reproductive technologies in the United States today. The report was written by an eleven-member committee, seven of whom are scientists and four of whom are not. Of the four nonscientists, the two lawyers on the committee, John Robertson and Lori Andrews, have been very public proponents of the new reproductive technologies.

In the initial part of the report, the committee defines its task as *supporting* the technologies: "Professional guidelines must not casually accede to restrictions on reproductive technologies that offer enhanced options. Rather, as this report attempts to do, guidelines should be set out that detail how the technologies may be offered with safety and ethical appropriateness. . . ."[51] Among the procedures the committee found ethical are: IVF; IVF using donor eggs, donor sperm, and donor embryos; artificial insemination with certification standards; patenting of instruments, products, and devices used in reproductive technologies; and embryo research when conducted "for the purpose of generating new knowledge not otherwise obtainable for benefiting human health."[52] As Gena Corea has noted, the only reservation it expressed was

> not for the physicians who are experimenting on women with risky procedures that studies show seldom work, but for women. The Committee castigates self-indulgent women who, to preserve their figures, might some day want to hire surrogate wives. (No such women have been heard from so far).[53]

Nowhere in this report are feminist objections to the technologies and to surrogacy noted, yet the committee did acknowledge religious objections.

Newspapers dutifully covered the report's contents, many with front page articles hailing its goals. *USA Today* reported that the American Fertility Society's recommendations "are the first attempt by leading experts to grapple with the complex ethical, medical and legal issues raised by the new ways to have babies."[54] No journalist noted that this was an in-house report that claimed to be much more than that or that seven of the official experts on the committee are themselves involved in the development and application of these technologies and two others are legal advocates of these procedures. The press covered the American Fertility Society's ethics report as if it were crafted by an impartial committee and no vested interests were involved.

Thus the new reproductive technologies were mediated as ethical by in-house experts who became in-house ethicists. There was the appearance of balance by including out-of-house lawyers and two professional ethicists on the committee. The inclusion of outside experts, most of whom agree with the in-house promoters, helped stifle doubt and skepticism. The experts orchestrated a chorus of self-promotion that squelched any opposition to new reproductive technologies and contracts as antitechnology.

Technology as Antiscience

The so-called progress of science is not only publicity driven but also technology driven. Scientists have been fond of retaining a distinction between science and technology that goes something like this: science is a particular way of knowing or body of knowledge, and technology is a particular kind of practice. Yet the reason for science's public success was its ability to produce technology. "The proof is in the pudding," or as Langdon Winner has phrased it, "The popular proof of science is technology. This is why we consider Bacon prophetic, Paracelsus quaint."[55] Therefore, Jacques Ellul and others have pointed out that there is no longer any meaningful distinction between science and technique;[56] what passes for science has become so thoroughly technologized that it is now driven by a need for innovative technologies, which is a form of technological determinism. Since science has gone to Wall Street and the U.S. Patent Office, not to mention the corporate and governmental grants that keep certain research results flowing, the ideal of science as a way of knowing, a free flow of ideas, and an open community of exchange has become arcane.

University science faculty have consulting arrangements with industry, and growing numbers of them have equity (ownership) positions in corporate ventures. "In 1984, nearly half of all biotechnology companies in the United States provided some kind of funding for university-based genetic engineering research."[57] Add to this the notion of "intellectual property" in the form of patenting of "new life forms," and the distinction between science and technology collapses all the more. It is no longer curiosity that propels science but the future technology of new commercial possibilities and products. "A government study of over 100 cooperative university-industry research projects found that industry and university scientists both ranked development of 'patentable products' as the most important goal of their joint research."[58]

In this so-called scientific climate, *it is technology that has become antiscience.* Technology has swallowed up science, abrogating its autonomous ways of knowing. *The problem is not one of dissidents being antitechnology but of technology being antiscience,* cutting off the independent spirit of scientific inquiry and shackling science to profitable techniques. In the same way, *many scientists have become antiscience* in that their work is directed toward producing technical products rather than exploring and expanding the parameters of scientific knowledge. As ties with industry increase, as equity positions are accepted, and as scientific products become patented, the number of independent scientists dwindles and scientific discovery is made more dependent on technological results.

Feminist critics of reproductive technologies contend that there is far too much technologized intervention into women's bodies. Too often, technological solutions leave women ravaged, as with fertility drugs and IVF. Reproduction is not fundamentally an issue of technology. Women may benefit from a genuine reproductive *science,* defined in the broadest sense of the term *science,* which does not necessarily mean more technology. Rather, real reproductive science may mean a more specific yet expansive knowledge of women's bodies with an emphasis on appropriate technology.

A genuine science puts its knowledge in context, not outside it. Technology is one aspect of this context. Thus genuine science is ecological, in the sense of recognizing that everything is related to everything else. In its original meaning and practice, science incorporates a wisdom of values, priorities, and limits. This is as intrinsic to the scientific task as its empirical methods.

The value of a technology must be judged not only by its consequences but by its purposes and the means it uses to achieve these.
While it is true that a technology can have unintended consequences,
the history of estrogen replacement therapy and other techniques emphasizes a more intentional part of the technological story. Many of
their negative consequences were forecast, but the forecasters were not
heeded. This history appears to be repeating itself in the widening use
of fetal reduction.

Fetal Reduction: A Case Study in
Reproductive Medical Progress

Many women begin the IVF journey with painful infertility workups.
They proceed to superovulation with powerful and dangerous fertility
drugs such as Pergonal and Clomid, and then doctors implant multiple
embryos in their uteri to ensure that at least one "takes." For some of
these women, the end product of the in vitro procedure is "fetal reduction" or "selective termination of pregnancy" or, in its kindler and gentler idiom, "selective continuation of pregnancy."

Fetal reduction is a technique used to decrease the number of
fetuses in utero of women on IVF programs who have become pregnant
with multiple embryos. Multiple embryos often result when women are
given fertility drugs and/or are implanted with a number of embryos
during the IVF procedure. If a woman becomes multiply pregnant, fertility specialists advise selective termination of some of these embryos
during the first trimester of pregnancy when fetal size is about one and
a half inches long. Guided by ultrasound, the doctor inserts a needle
filled with potassium chloride into the fetal chest cavity, causing death
by heart failure. The fetus is eventually absorbed by the woman's body.

The media discusses the ethics of fetal reduction as if the critical
issue is one of the morality of abortion, not the morality of using powerful fertility drugs on women or the ethics of implanting multiple
embryos to begin with. For example, a 1988 front page *New York Times*
article on fetal reduction bore the headline: "Multiple Fetuses Raise
New Issues Tied to Abortion." The headline more accurately should
have read: "Multiple Fetuses Raise New Issues Tied to Fertility Drugs
and Multiple Embryo Implants."

Multiple implants and superovulation are more examples of another so-called miracle technology gone wrong. Fetal reduction is another technical fix launched as a corrective to a past technical fix that has failed. Yet few see the absurdity of treating one disaster with another. Infertility drugs, multiple embryo implants, and their recent accomplice, fetal reduction, are new iatrogenic "diseases," where the supposed cure (fertility drugs and multiple implants) produces affliction (multiple pregnancies, all of which cannot be sustained) and where the so-called side effect (multiple embryos) is more accurately a frequent *effect* of the treatment. The morbid risks of fetal reduction are many. Women can start bleeding or develop infections, causing them danger, premature labor, and the loss of all the fetuses. Uterine bleeding can cause irreparable neurological damage to any fetuses that remain after others are "reduced."

These new reproductive technologies perpetuate a self-reinforcing loop of destructive feedback. This destructive feedback is built right into the medical-technical endeavor of superovulation and/or multiple implants. Trumpeted as treatments for infertility, procedures such as IVF and superovulatory drugs are now becoming the new pathogens leading to more bodily intervention, invasiveness, morbidity, and experimentation on women.

Moreover, the popular media often portray women as the instigators and motivators of the fetal reduction procedure. Women are represented as demanding fetal reduction. An article in the *Daily Mail* phrased it this way:

> A woman carrying five babies [*sic*] after hormone treatment for infertility *became distressed* and sought to end the pregnancy. Surgeons *compromised*. They sacrificed the lives of three ten-week-old embryos and the 34-year-old woman went on to give birth to healthy twin girls.[59]

Thus women are portrayed as emotional and exacting, and the doctors are pictured as conceding to their demands. The irrational woman is saved by the rationality of the benevolent doctors who effect a technological "compromise" with her implied extravagant request. There is no mention of the irrationality of a procedure that is problematic at its core and that requires another problematic procedure as a corrective.

As philosopher Christine Overall has pointed out, "Women's so-called 'demand' for selective termination of pregnancy is not a primordial expression of individual need, but a socially constructed response to prior medical interventions."[60] Overall recognizes that selective termination is a technology that generates a problem as a so-called solution to another problem. But she defends the continued availability of fetal reduction based on the fact that a medical system that causes multiple problem pregnancies has the responsibility to provide women with a "potential, if flawed response."[61] It is much better, however, to advocate for an end to technologies that generate more problems and provoke more of their own pathologies.

Nonetheless, the media perpetuate the image of fetal reduction as a miracle technology. In 1988 *People* magazine ran a story called, "A Dramatic Medical Rescue Saves the Schellin Twins from Their Mother's Nightmare Pregnancy." Beth Schellin conceived nine embryos after being treated with the fertility drug Pergonal. After one fetus had miscarried, six were selectively terminated, and the two remaining fetuses, later born, were portrayed as "the survivors of an operation at the very frontier of reproductive medicine." In keeping with its heroic portrait, the procedure was called "prenatal triage."[62] And in keeping with the dubious way that women are depicted, the article's headline played up the pregnancy, *not* the fertility drugs and/or multiple implants, as a nightmare.

This same article was accompanied by a box insert that headlined the fear that "Selective Termination May Be Abused." It raised ethical questions such as, Who decides which fetus is terminated and which survives? Could the procedure be used for sex predetermination to save a male fetus at the expense of "reducing" a female? And ironically, Could fetal reduction be used as a "remedy for incompetent practices at fertility clinics"? The point seems lost on the questioner that superovulation and multiple implants that generate multiple pregnancies are incompetent to begin with. Even a Catholic theologian, Richard McCormick, defended selective termination as "a lifesaving intervention, an alternative to letting all the fetuses die," without commenting on the interventions that spawned the need for selective termination. Taking the defense strategy even further, Dr. Mark Evans, a specialist in multiple pregnancies, argued that fetal reduction is not an abortion.

"The goal of an abortion is to end the pregnancy. . . . Here the woman desperately wants a child but is in a situation where she would not have any children without selective termination."[63]

Discussing fetal reduction as a solution for problem pregnancies produced by fertility drugs and multiple implants once more takes the focus off the self-interest of the medical scientists. Fetal reduction was launched to increase the number of IVF pregnancies, thus boosting their abysmal success rates. As with fetal reduction, the continuing development of new reproductive technologies drives the supposed need for scores of other reproductive technologies to offset the first action/reaction. What is the price of this medical progress if it leaves women with an increased dependency on more and more problematical technical solutions? In considering the in vitro process from start to finish, we must recognize that sectors of women have almost no control over their own processes of conception, pregnancy, and birth. And many women are being violated repeatedly by these procedures in the belief that such drugs and procedures are their salvation. At what cost have these medical advances been implemented, and how many more of these reproductive procedures will be generated before there is even some modest realization of the necessity for limits?

The Necessity for Limits

The necessity for limits has been a forceful tenet in environmental circles. Recycling, reusing, and reducing waste, with the emphasis on not generating problematic products to begin with, have been crucial to the present current of environmental activism. Would that the same commitment to prohibiting problematic drugs and technologies were prevalent in the reproductive realm. As environmental engineer H. Patricia Hynes has noted, toxic reproductive chemicals are exempted from an environmental consciousness: "As a wave of green lifestyle washes over industrial countries, making people conscious of not putting any unnecessary synthetic chemical substances on and into their body, why are women being advised to use synthethic hormones?"[64] Further, why is there an unmitigated increase in the number and kinds of drugs and technical fixes that are being prescribed for women—especially in the reproductive realm—at a time when the rest of the planet is being warned about the risks of chemical and technical fixes? Can we be disturbed about chemically fed plants and animals and remain unconcerned about chemically fed women, many of whom take scores of drugs from menstruation to menopause?

Are women being exempted from the natural world as more and more bodily processes become subject to the medicalization of technical progress? Surely, a genuine ecological consciousness should spot this glaring pollution of women. If environmentalists are quick to recognize the mechanizing of nature, why are they so slow to recognize the pathologizing of women's natural bodily processes? Why are synthetic and technical procedures being limited on plants and animals, yet being increased on women?

Environmentalism has increased consciousness of the limits of the ecosystem. The necessity of limits has also been raised in medical-ethical circles. Much of this debate was initiated with the publication of Daniel Callahan's book, *What Kind of Life? The Limits of Medical Progress,* in which he talks about medical and human priorities and the American unwillingness to set limits on medical interventions.[65] The debate about the limits of medical interventions and innovations has also been raised in legislatures and health-financing contexts, as federal, state, and private health providers wrestle with decisions about how much and what kind of health care and techniques to cover. Yet many state and federal bills seem bent on expanding, rather than limiting, coverage for costly high-tech procedures such as technological reproduction.

In 1987, Massachusetts signed into law a bill that would require insurance companies to pay for the medical treatment of infertility. Although this law is not yet implemented, it covers all aspects of diagnosis and treatment of infertility, including superovulation, in vitro fertilization, and embryo transfer. Earlier, Maryland passed a law that extended coverage to in vitro fertilization. And more recently, Hawaii and Texas have laws requiring insurance coverage of infertility procedures.

On the federal level, Representative Pat Schroeder has introduced a bill into Congress covering many aspects of women's health and reproductive services. Launched in the midst of the repressive contraceptive and abortion climate in the United States, especially in the aftermath of the 1989 Supreme Court decision on abortion, the purpose of

H.R. 1161 is to offset this climate by promoting "greater equity in the delivery of health care services to American women through expanded research on women's health issues, improved access to health care services, and the development of disease prevention activities responsive to the needs of women."[66]

Many parts of this legislation are excellent and much needed, such as research into contraception for men and improved barrier methods such as diaphragms and condoms. However, along with these laudatory provisions, this legislation requires insurance programs for federal workers to cover "family building" expenses such as infertility treatments, "including procedures to achieve pregnancy and procedures to carry pregnancy to term."[67]

With Representative Olivia Snowe as cosponsor, Schroeder has also built into this bill an appropriation request for 75 million dollars to set up five federal centers to conduct research into birth control and fertility. This section, entitled the "Contraceptive and Infertility Research Centers Act," provides for continued research "for the purpose of diagnosing and treating infertility." Schroeder has said that this would cover IVF research as well as "clinical trials of new or improved drugs and devices for the diagnosis and treatment of infertility in both males and females."[68] Since no technologies or drugs are detailed in this section, it is difficult to know what specific research and technologies would be investigated. However, one thing is certain: if IVF is an intended part of the research and of proposed federal workers' health coverage, federal funding will be used for research and coverage of an experimental and debilitating technology for women. And instead of recognizing the need to limit costly and experimental research and treatments that serve the few, this legislation will promote medical expansionism over the lives and bodies of women.

The United States is not alone in this debate about insurance coverage of new reproductive technologies such as in vitro fertilization. Other countries have been more critical and controlling of high technologies. Australia has begun to survey the costs of burgeoning high technologies and drugs, and in 1988 the Australian Family Association called for ending Medicare benefits for in vitro fertilization. The secretary of the association, Michael Barr, pointed out that each live birth by IVF costs $40,500 Australian dollars. Other governmental groups and individuals called for a review of the cost-efficiency of such procedures and blamed increased coverage of high-tech procedures for "health care cost blow-out."

At an Anglo-American conference on biomedical ethics, ethicist Arthur Caplan noted that the usual measure employed by insurers to evaluate a treatment's efficacy is a 50 percent success rate over a five-year period, based on the performance of all providers. In no country of the world does IVF technology fulfill this standard of efficacy.[69] The question is, then, why should it be insured? Additionally, technologies, such as in vitro fertilization, are promoted as cures for infertility when, in reality, they do nothing to treat infertility. They may provide some very few people with biological children but they do *not* alleviate infertility.

More important, in the reproductive context, certain desires have been transformed into needs. The desire for a child, for example, has been represented as a need of supposedly infertile couples. As science invents new needs for people, often people who can pay and who are of the right race, sex, class, ability, or sexual preference, the critical health needs of most people go unattended and uncovered by medical insurance.

Although usually framed in economic terms, the issue of limits is much more than economic cost containment. Progress cannot simply be equated with the unlimited development and application of more reproductive technologies. We must pay attention to the values and circumstances surrounding their use. For example, when surrogacy promotes a class of women who can be bought and sold as breeders, is it really progress that more supposedly infertile couples can have babies in this way? Progress for whom?

Reproduction is on the frontier of an endless technical and medical horizon, where we could simply spend more and more money, intervening in the bodily processes of more and more women at great cost to women's health and well-being and at the expense of providing for the genuine need of others for basic health care and delivery, but doing nothing to improve human life. The increased medicalization and technologizing of reproduction is part of the debate over the limits of medical progress and the concomitant necessity for limiting what insurance coverage can pay for. We cannot continue to develop these technologies with a total indifference to any kind of limits and priorities.

These limits and priorities should be measured by many things. First, since women are the primary "patients" in this realm of reproductive techniques, the primary question is, Do these technologies benefit *women*—nôt only individual women but women as a social group? Second, limits and priorities should be measured by reference to what is happening in other areas of health care. There is a crisis in AIDS women and babies; one out of eight women suffers from breast cancer; and the U.S. maternal morbidity and infant mortality rates, as compared with those of other industrial countries, are high. These deaths often take place in the same hospitals where elite reproductive technologies are being developed and expanded for the select few who have access to them. For African Americans, the neonatal death rate is more than twice the national average, and for Native Americans the neonatal death rate is five times the national average. The issue should not be increasing access to experimental, costly, and debilitating technologies but rather implementing priorities that prevent maternal morbidity and infant mortality as well as ensure basic access to nutrition, sanitation, prenatal care, and prevention of disease. Some will say that these reproductive technologies need not be pitted against access to basic health needs. Yet these technologies can only be defended in the interests of servicing the few, not the many others whose pressing needs go unmet because research and money are siphoned off in the quest for more profitable and high technologies of reproduction.

The development of more reproductive drugs and technologies is not in keeping with an ecology of women's health. The marketing of medical progress through new reproductive technologies assures continued experimentation on women's bodies and a spiraling of the cycle in which women are encouraged to try every new sickening and debilitating technique or drug, hyped as the next miracle cure, to have a child. Progress ultimately is a moral, social, and political standard not measured by increased medical-technical innovation. When the fullness of this standard is ignored, and when science and technology separate themselves from this standard, progress is a form of social self-deception. The corrective to this limited standard of progress cannot come from more reproductive technology but from a progress that ensures the welfare, not of women only as individuals, but of all women in all areas of the world.

CHAPTER FIVE

The International Traffic
in Women, Children,
and Fetuses

New reproductive procedures have helped spawn an international reproductive trafficking in women, children, and fetuses that is largely unrecognized. Unlike the trafficking in drugs, which conjures up a sensational scenario of a vast criminal underworld, few associate the technologically sophisticated and medicalized world of new reproductive arrangements with international trafficking.

Trafficking involves an exchange. The key object of reproductive trafficking is women and what issues from their bodies; the subject or agents of this exchange are mostly men and what issues from their genes, their research and experimentation, their money, and their interventions. Men, whether as doctors, lawyers, brokers, or sperm sources, are the traffickers, the go-betweens, who carry on the exchange in women's bodies for surrogate contracts, women's eggs for use in IVF, and women's embryos for use in embryo experimentation and fetal tissue exchange.

Reproductive traffic often crosses international borders. International adoption arrangements in which children are procured from women for a price or simply taken are a prevalent form of reproductive trafficking. There is also an alleged traffic in children for organ export. And a traffic in fetal tissue has been reported from abroad. However, trafficking in women, children, and fetuses need not cross international borders. Surrogate arrangements are part of a national traffic in women used for various reproductive purposes and are accepted as technological progress and reproductive freedom in the United States.

The idea of trafficking captures crucial but usually unobserved elements of technological and contractual reproduction: the import and export of eggs, fetal tissue, drugs, and technologies; the commerce of buying and selling bodies, body parts, and bodily capacities; the dealings between individuals and groups, even within the international medical research community; the brokering through international reproductive networks; and the passengers or cargo carried by a particular transport system (women, fetuses, and children). It is the reality of reproductive trafficking that establishes the connections between adoption, surrogacy, and medical research.

The consumers of women's reproductive faculties and functions have language and meaning on their side, a language and meaning that distract from the trafficking inherent in technological and contractual reproduction. For example, many commentators have noted that the term *surrogate mother* carries all the negative connotations of reproductive contracts, thereby masking the male demand for genetic progeny, the professionals who carry out the procedures, and the brokers who mediate the contracts and benefit most by this enterprise. "No expression specifically designates the sires; the initiators and principal beneficiaries of birth contracts float in the carefree realm of the unnamed. . . . Safely hidden by the discourse, as if they themselves were 'carried' by the bearing mothers, these men vanish from the linguistic context, and their motivations, their interests, and their roles are thereby easily concealed."[1]

Trafficking wrenches the term *surrogate mother* out of its present context of blaming women and highlights that women are the objects of international exchange. Trafficking situates surrogate arrangements in the system of gender inequality—as a practice that enhances the subordination of women by making women into reproductive objects of global exchange.

The idea and the reality of trafficking cut through a Western culture of liberal individualism in which procreative liberty and reproductive freedom reign as the ethical and legal principles governing reproductive arrangements; where the woman's body and the child that may result are seen as property to be contracted for or "given" within a family context; and where surrogate reproduction is featured as a triumph of science and technique. Trafficking challenges the notion that surrogacy is a financial alternative for women, highlights the economic reality that brokers take the largest share of the profit, and spotlights the international networks of technological reproduction.

Much of the opposition to reproductive technologies and arrangements has obscured the sex-dominated social subordination of women by focusing on what is done to fetuses and children. Many well-meaning opponents of technological reproduction are quick to defend children and children's rights, thereby making the violation one of the exploitation of children and discounting similar abuses to adult women. Separating the exploitation of children, however, from the exploitation of women conveys the impression that it is tolerable to use women in reproductive technologies and contracts, whereas the use of children is indefensible. Children are perceived as having no choice; women are perceived as choosing.

It is necessary not only to insist that the exploitation of women is inextricably linked to the exploitation of children, but also to show how the trafficking in children for sexual and reproductive purposes is the end result of the trafficking in women. New reproductive technologies and contracts only add to this overall organized structure of the sexual and reproductive trafficking in women and children worldwide.

Connecting Sexual and Reproductive Trafficking

Reproductive trafficking can be compared to the sexual trafficking in women that is currently established in various parts of the world.[2] Take the geographical region of Asia, for example. At least 700,000 women are in prostitution in Bangkok today, 30,000 of whom are estimated to be under sixteen. In Korea and the Philippines, there are hundreds of thousands more. Eunice Kim, a human rights activist who is president of the Korea chapter of Asia Women United, claims that there are a million prostitutes in South Korea out of a population of 41 million. In Korea, the government does little to enforce the law against prostitution and has encouraged prostitution to lure foreign businessmen and trade.[3] The Korean government has even glorified the role of women in the sex tourism industry as service to the nation.

Why so many prostitutes? Many of these women have been re-cruited for the American military—more recently in the Philippines, yesterday in Vietnam and Korea—and for a burgeoning pornography and sex tourism industry that has been imported from the West and Japan. Combine this with a documented and burgeoning "mail order" bride industry,[4] and it is not a far reach to a "mail order" baby industry where women are bought and sold as breeders.

Many women in prostitution, for example in Korea during the war, became pregnant by foreign soldiers who were stationed there. The rest and recreation areas set up by the U.S. military and the prostitution mills they created left many women with a legacy of more than sexual exploitation. They left them with children. Other women engaged in sexual activity with soldiers on the promise of a marriage that never occurred. When the soldiers left, the businessmen entered, having a ready-made set-up for the sex tourism industry. In addition, prejudice against unwed mothers and so-called illegitimate children, combined with prejudice against children of mixed blood, caused many children to be abandoned and many women to become vulnerable to sexual and reproductive trafficking.

The extent to which reproductive trafficking is linked with actual sex trafficking networks is unknown and has not been addressed in news accounts or studies. But in South America and Sri Lanka, women have been procured specifically for breeding purposes. A 1986 *Sunday Herald* news article from Australia reported, "Several women plucked from the Colombo slums by baby 'farmers' have claimed they were forced to sleep with European tourists so the babies they produced would be fairer skinned, more appealing to Western couples and, there-fore, more valuable."[5] In 1982 the report of the Anti-Slavery Society for the Protection of Human Rights, prepared for the United Nations Working Group on Slavery, stated that the Sri Lankan deputy minister of social services had evidence of organized "baby farms" that ensured a supply of salable children to foreigners. Evidence of a particular con-nection of child trafficking between Switzerland and Sri Lanka was also reported in which Swiss buyers paid up to 10,000 Swiss francs for a baby, the bulk of the payment going to the brokers involved.[6]

The same 1986 *Sunday Herald* article reported that "baby farms" were secretly established in Sri Lanka, each stocked with twenty or more pregnant women. Once the mothers gave birth, their children were taken away to privately operated children's homes, where the owners or free-lance baby brokers struck deals with would-be adoptive parents, especially from Australia.[7] Local Sri Lankan newspapers contained accounts of a "baby mafia" that issued death threats to critics of the trade. Vinitha Jayasinghe, commissioner of childcare in Sri Lanka, said, "We know many local women carry either their own babies or someone else's, leaving the country for various reasons."[8] Jayasinghe and other officials believe the trade involves hotel operators, doctors, lawyers, and corrupt officials who bring in foreign couples, sell them babies, and then arrange legal adoptions, with 1,500 babies leaving the island each year as part of such adoption schemes.[9]

In 1988 the Guatemalan Parliament expressed concern over the business of baby selling, noting especially the ways in which women were being used to breed children for others. Governmental minister Roberto Valle confirmed a new wave of complaints about "gestation houses" in which women agree to get pregnant and give up the child for an amount of money. These children were then reported sold to Europeans and North Americans.[10]

Adoption can become a form of reproductive trafficking as well. Evidence of adoption trafficking exists in North America, although trafficking is more difficult to organize within these borders. A Canadian journal found one U.S. lawyer on the West Coast who located young unwed mothers, encouraged them to have their babies on a Caribbean "baby farm," all expenses paid, and then placed their babies with adoptive couples back in the States.[11] Private adoptions have always been vulnerable to exploitation because they are largely unregulated, and the lawyer's role in these adoptions is a gray area.[12] Many lawyers exploit the fine line between baby brokering and networking for people wanting to adopt.[13] With the increased legalization of private adoptions in many states, this line will be blurred further as lawyers take on (for profit) the role religious and public agency personnel once performed.[14] Because there is widespread abuse, organizations such as the Child Welfare League are calling for an end to all private adoptions. "Many adoption experts say private adoptions leave children at risk, birth mothers with too little or no preparation for the consequences of their decision and adoptive parent open to huge bills even when no baby ends up in their arms."[15]

Internationally, another facet of the traffic in women includes the selling of female fetuses while they are still in the womb. In India, a 1986 study by the Joint Women's Programme documented that parents are selling unborn female children into prostitution. The study is believed to be the most authoritative and reliable report on prostitution in India, documenting the situation in twelve of India's twenty-three states and two federally administered territories. The study claims that some deals are made when fetuses are three months old, commanding a price of 3,500 rupees. When born, most of these girl children are sold into prostitution.[16] Joint Women's Programme spokeswoman Jyotsna Chatterjee said that "women are sold like cheese."[17]

The children of women in prostitution are numerous—probably five million in India alone. A high proportion of these children also end up in prostitution.[18] Thus we have here the literal reproduction of prostitution in which prostitutes are used to perpetuate the institution through the sexual exploitation of their children. Dutch Labor member of Parliament Piet Stoffelen, in a comprehensive report linking adoption, prostitution, pornography, and slavery to the traffic in children from developing countries to the U.S. and Europe, documents that prostitutes most in demand are between the ages of ten and fourteen: "The prices for the different kinds of prostitution with children are much higher than with adult prostitutes (for instance five times the 'adult price')." And, "Over the years, the prostitution of minors has become an industry, one from which many families make their entire living."[19] Most important to recognize, however, is that "child prostitution is part of the overall structure [of organized prostitution], not an institution apart."[20] Dr. Atilio Alvarez, an Argentinian expert in issues of child justice, also connects the illegal traffic in children to organ traffic, slave labor, and the traffic in women for prostitution.[21]

Surrogacy is becoming part of the global traffic in women, since brokers are tapping into the international supply and demand. Surrogate brokers advertise abroad for buyers who cannot obtain a legal surrogate in their own countries. Noel Keane, the notorious U.S. surrogate broker, attempted to establish a surrogate agency in Frankfurt, Germany, but was rebuffed by a coalition of opponents, including many feminist groups. Called United Family International, Keane's agency had supplied American women to men from France, Italy, Israel, Greece, and Australia before a German court ordered its closing.[22] Moreover, as surrogacy is increasingly combined with other new reproductive technologies, as in surrogate gestation, where the so-called surrogate's own eggs are not used and where she serves as a mere environment for growing the fetus, the number of women used in systems of surrogacy will expand. John Stehura, president of the Bionetics Foundation, which hires women for surrogate arrangements, maintains that the standard U.S. rate of 10,000 dollars is too high a price for couples to pay for renting a womb. Once so-called surrogates can be culled from developing countries where poor women will supposedly leap at the chance to earn, say, 5,000 dollars, the surrogate industry can increase internationally.[23]

We must look at the global network of relations that govern surrogate arrangements and connect surrogacy with the entire reproductive traffic in women and children. Unfortunately, what happens to women and children in many developing countries is deeply exacerbated by the U.S. liberal attitude toward prostitution, pornography, and surrogacy. The United States has exported the image of surrogacy, as well as that of prostitution and pornography, as *work* done by happy and altruistic women who do it not only for the money but for the joy they give to others. This liberalism, called reproductive choice, masks the systematic and organized nature of an international industry that traffics in the bodies of women. And it has little concern for the effects of such pseudochoices on women worldwide.

The extolling of surrogacy as a right is in the worst tradition of both U.S. individualism and U.S. isolationism, because it makes no connection between how such a supposed right will affect women's rights in the West and women's rights around the world. It is only by making international connections that we see that reproductive trafficking is linked with sexual trafficking worldwide—prostitution with surrogacy, sexual exploitation with adoption.

International Adoption

As I investigated the international dimensions of surrogacy (what brokers call intrauterine adoption), it became clear that an established reproductive traffic—the international adoption trade—already prevailed that surrogacy would only enhance. International adoption has become a human rights issue only recently. The benevolent picture of Westerners giving a home to abandoned, undernourished, and uncared-for children from developing countries obscures the real way in which children have often been procured for adoptions. For too long, adoption has been seen as a welfare issue—taking children away from supposedly bad homes or no homes and giving them good homes. Within this framework, adopting parents are viewed as saviors. Yet many prospective parents never ask where the children come from or how they got from there to here. Other would-be parents, who may know about the origins of the child's procurement for adoption, reason that children are better off with them. For the most part, however, many assume that adoptable children arrive via legitimate routes.

Procurement happens in different ways. As with sexual trafficking, the flow of the reproductive trafficking in women and children moves from Third World to First World countries. Much of this trafficking is, in fact, directly linked to so-called *development*. The main child-importing countries are the United States, Canada, and many European countries, especially Sweden, Denmark, the Netherlands, Italy, and France. In addition to Korea, the main child-exporting nations are in Latin America. From 1975 to 1980, 90 percent of the children adopted from abroad came from Asia and Latin America.[24]

In 1987 foreign adoptees were reported to be arriving in the United States at the rate of one child every forty-eight minutes.[25] Many of these children traditionally came from Asian countries such as Korea; although adoptions from Korea have decreased, it remains by far the main adoption resource of the world.[26] Thailand has also been a major supplier of adoptable children. The Bangkok-based Centre for the Protection of Children's Rights issued a report in 1987 contending that six thousand Thai children had been abducted in Thailand and smuggled across the border into Malaysia since 1981, bound not only for Malaysia but for Europe.[27] *South* magazine reported that most of these six thousand children were bought from prostitutes.[28] And the Anti-Slavery Society documented that many of these same children were intercepted and returned to the Southern Thailand Provincial Welfare Office to be cared for.[29]

Within the last ten years Latin America has become another major supplier of adoptable children to the developed world, particularly to the United States. As in Korea, the exporting of children from Latin America to the United States has been going on for as long as the U.S. has been politically and militarily involved in the area.

A primary cause of the trafficking in women and children for adoption—both legal and illegal—is the ravaging of countries by U.S.-supported military and civilian governments. The creation of massive-scale refugee camps in El Salvador, for example, is the tragic consequence of U.S.-backed civil war. Prostitution and abandoned children are two of the least-talked-about results of militarism.[30] With war comes the war against women—rape. Unwanted pregnancies from rape by Guatemalan soldiers is one of the three major products of militaristic violence in the Guatemalan highlands.[31] Soldiers are often paid for bringing babies and orphans back to the barracks and passing them on to illegal adoption networks.

The outcrop of U.S. involvement in Central America—in Honduras, Guatemala, and El Salvador—has traditionally been exportable products such as coffee and fruit. Now women and children have become the most recent cash crops, for sexual and reproductive purposes. In Guatemala, for example, the exporting of children has become the "primary nontraditional product" of the country. These were the words used by Mario Taracena, Guatemalan Congressman and president of the Commission to Protect Children,[32] who also asserted that Guatemala receives more than 20 million dollars annually in profits from the sale of this "product." Taking the region as a whole, "Latin America ranks first in the sale of children to foreigners."[33]

Not all of these children are orphans, nor do many of the children pass through reputable adoption agencies. Many are so-called black market babies procured by brokers—local lawyers or other businessmen linked to the same kind of brokers in the North. Some lawyers create their own procurement networks, hiring scouts who scavenge the villages, the refugee camps, cities, and hospitals for children. These middlemen persuade destitute women to give up their babies, and they pay what is often a pittance to mothers who are in dire need of money and guilt-ridden because they cannot provide, care for, and feed the children.[34] In one refugee camp in El Salvador, women reportedly told visitors that strange men talked them into giving over some of their children. "He said he had a friend who would send them to a rich country and they would be better off,"[35] one woman told a reporter.

Close scrutiny of Guatemalan adoption lists by human rights groups reveals that it is always the same lawyers who broker adoptions abroad. The International Federation for Human Rights found that these lawyers even specialized in adoption to a given country.[36] Their report also mentions that the American Embassy in Guatemala is the only embassy of a Western country, as of 1988, to refuse adoption emanating from lawyers known for their involvement in illegal practices. Certainly, this is the right course of action, but many other countries also need to register their refusals.

Increasingly, many children who end up on the legal and illegal adoption circuit are stolen from maternity wards in hospitals by doctors, nurses, or other personnel who tell mothers that their babies died in childbirth. In Turkey, doctors have given false death certificates for babies and shipped the babies off to northern Europe. Lawyers also pay off hospital workers to bring them babies, some left behind in maternity wards. Birth certificates and other papers are falsified, with government officials often taking part in this process.[37]

The International Federation for Human Rights sent a mission of investigators to Haiti and Guatemala in 1988. They reported that the key to facilitating adoption trafficking "consists only in giving a newborn child a false identity, and then following the regular [adoption] procedure. The establishment of the birth certificate is the most important and, at the same time, the aspect of the adoption procedure where falsification is easiest."[38] Thus many adoptions that end up as legal in the North may actually begin as illegal in the South. Once a child is given a fabricated identity, the whole adoption procedure can be perfectly regularized.

Kidnappings account for many of these supposedly adoptable children, not only from hospitals but from women's arms. Other children have been snatched from their beds by organized bands of kidnappers.[39] Many children also are picked from the streets and lumped into a category of "abandoned" children, most of whom are not truly abandoned. The NGO (Non-Governmental Organization) *Forum* distinguishes between children *on* the street, children *of* the street, and abandoned children. As of 1984, it was estimated that there were 170 million abandoned/street children worldwide. However, 61 percent of this total earn a living *on* the street and maintain regular contact with their families, while 32 percent are children *of* the street who, for the most part, live independently but have sporadic family contact. Only seven percent have been, strictly speaking, abandoned.[40]

Brokers also take advantage of the stigma against single women with out-of-wedlock children. Independent of economic need, single women who get pregnant often give over babies for adoption. In cultures where religion and tradition deprive women of birth control and abortion and where nothing is demanded of the father for his responsibility in producing a child, children are ripe for export.

As the demand for babies in the North increases, brokers have resorted to paying teenage girls to get pregnant. In Honduras, for example, such girls are reportedly kept under surveillance by brokers to monitor their eating habits and prenatal care.[41] In Brazil, a country with much racial diversity, networks of brokers offer satisfaction for every type of child demanded—most of them light skinned. Light-skinned babies are plentiful in Argentina as well, where 90 percent of the population is of European descent and where blond-haired, blue-eyed babies are in especially high demand.[42] In Brazil "reproductive teams," often composed of lawyers, doctors, nurses, scouts, and other middlemen, contract with light-skinned women to bear children for foreign men or couples,[43] a practice not so different from surrogacy in the North.

The Stoffelen Report on the *Traffic in Children* prepared for the Council of Europe (see note 19), claims that aid agencies sometimes operate as covers for adoption trafficking in women and children.[44] Such an agency is the model extolled by one surrogate broker in the United States. John Stehura, president of the Bionetics Foundation, projects setting up a surrogate agency in Mexico, specifically in Mexicali and Tijuana, fast-growing cities not far from the U.S border. In a 1987 interview conducted by Gena Corea, he volunteered his plans for customized surrogacy in Mexico:

> Stehura: Offer a medical clinic. Have a doctor come in once a week. Do all these U.S. charity-type things but direct it towards pregnancy and surrogacy.

Corea: So if you had a clinic where you had a doctor come in once a week, people would begin to trust that facility? Is that it?

Stehura: It might look something like a Children's Home Society which would be a non-profit type of adoption agency. . . . Very much like the food programs, like the medical aid programs where U.S. medical doctors go there on weekends—that sort of thing—to help in poor neighborhoods. So I would be literally mimicking something pretty much like that.[45]

In Stehura's words, "the proper presentation of surrogate parenting" in Mexico involves softening up the local women with free medical care in order to give them an incentive to undergo a surrogate pregnancy for a U.S. client. "You could devastate them with money and things. . . . It would save them 20 years of scratching." He particularly wants to make his surrogacy appeal to women for whom "the family linkage has broken down," those who can "appreciate their own independence."[46] His model is based on existing institutions that pose as charitable aid agencies, for example, for purposes of adoption, and that already have a preexisting system set up for a reproductive market in women and children.

It is not surprising that private aid agencies are involved in reproductive trafficking, since aid and aid agencies have been associated with other commercial and/or political purposes. For example, camps in Honduras for Nicaraguan refugees set up by various private U.S. rightwing groups and by the U.S. Agency for International Development (USAID) were consistently used as bases for producing men and children to fight for the contras.[47] In like manner, "officials of an agency offering relief in refugee camps in Bangladesh are in fact involved in trafficking in unaccompanied refugee children."[48]

Other methods also are used to procure women and children for adoptive purposes. Reports were published that authorities in Malaysia discovered six live babies packed into a suitcase being smuggled into the country from Thailand. The babies were bound for prospective parents in Europe and the United States.[49] Agencies operating out of Holland and Malta charge up to 5,000 dollars for a "service fee," often paid by frustrated affluent couples who are on long legal adoption waiting lists in their own countries. For this price and more, middlemen will search for babies for couples who come to them from all over Europe. Pieces of paper are given to the couple saying the birth mother agreed to the adoption. Additional charges for transportation, legal fees, traveling expenses, and supposed orphanage costs can push the total price tag to over 30,000 dollars.[50]

In India it is alleged that solicitors walk around airports with funny lumps, that is, babies, under their arms. In South Korea, it has been reported that women are returning yearly to private adoption agencies with a baby, picking up payment, and being cheerily waved off with a "see you next year."[51] In the news accounts, one hears a lot about "The Baby Trade," but one hears very little about how the babies are procured and much less about how the women are procured for purposes of the trade. But it is all of a piece. The same organized middlemen who procure babies procure women to have those babies.

Many discussions of international adoption focus only on the supply factor, but it is demand in this instance that creates supply. Dr. Ahilemah Jonet, a Malaysian lawyer working on the international legal aspects of the trafficking in children, points out that none of this supply of babies could exist without the demand for children in the North and West.

> Commentators propose reform in the law and procedure on adoption, or plead for a revised policy on intercountry adoption. They omit the examination of the source factor—the demand. . . . Consequently, the adoptive parents—the consumers—escape the blame as the innocent party.[52]

Children of international adoptions are also beginning to speak out on this subject. Writing from the perspective of a Korean woman who was adopted, Mi Ok Bruining challenges the stereotypes, myths, and lies of the international adoption industry. Speaking especially to white lesbians and gay men, she underscores the increasing popularity of international adoptions among lesbians and gays as a form of consumption where "children of color are the commodities and products and victims of ownership and living human property, and this process is being disguised as the desire to parent a child. . . ." Each time critics focus on the demand factor, thus linking the supply of international adoptees with the demand by Westerners for children, they are branded as enemies of the proadoption movement. "I have received hate mail, have been accused of being angry, mentally ill, and of having unresolved issues with my adoptive parents. I have been told that I am destroying the hope and future of adopted children, and I have also been condemned by a few adopted Korean adults."[53] Thus her challenge to and criticism of the social and political aspects of international adoptions is trivialized as unresolved personal problems with her own adoption.

Maria Josefina Becker, 1988 director of the Brazilian Federal Child Welfare Agency FUNABEM, puts the demand factor into institutional perspective:

> In practice, since the "demand" is greater than the "supply," one ends up looking for children to satisfy the needs of the couples or families wishing to adopt. To the extent that they actively undertake the search for children to be adopted, couples and agencies involved in international adoption, their generous and humane motives notwithstanding, increase the pressures favouring a rupture between the poor child and his or her family rather than strengthening the ties between them. These pressures are exercised on the family directly, through description of the paradise-like future (a perfect home in a country where poverty does not exist) that the parents will deny their child if they refuse to permit adoption. Not even the local official or private child welfare agencies are exempt from this pressure, when the sending of a child to a distant and idealised country is portrayed as an easy and more promising alternative to the creation and administration of family support programmes, an arduous task whose success will not always be evident in the short run. In this way conditions encouraging the *"production" of abandonment* are created, apparently motivated by the assistance and protection of the child, but which in reality serve the interests of the adoptive parents.[54]

International demand and the many foreign agencies and individuals vying with each other for securing children from abroad check the possibilities for women and children finding resources in their own countries. Because of the pressing demand for intercountry adoption, children are often hastily routed along international adoptive highways.

This pressing demand, however, is for white babies. Although we hear much about the shortage of babies for the two million Americans who at any given time are looking to adopt, the shortage is of babies who are as close to white as possible. Racism prompts would-be parents systematically to seek out light-skinned children from Asia and South and

Central America. Jonet points out that this popularity of light-skinned babies is not confined to the West but is increasingly prevalent in Third World countries. She cites her own country, Malaysia, as an example of a preference for light-complexioned Thai adoptees, preferably female, who are viewed as well mannered, hardworking, and obedient.[55]

Adoptive parents also talk about international adoption as a noble act, as rescuing children from poverty and misery. They envision themselves as making some dent in the problem of world poverty, a dent, however, "which does not require any major changes in lifestyle." Jonet views this as a romantic route, "a poor child of another race, from a far away place is an exotic souvenir to take home when one visits the country as a tourist."[56] For many adoptive parents, adopting a light-skinned child from a foreign country also eliminates the possibility of the natural parent(s) returning to claim the child.

Of course, many persons wanting to adopt sincerely desire to be good parents, but personal goodwill is not the only issue here. We must place the discussion of intercountry adoption in a social and political context and acknowledge that much more is at stake than a personal goal to parent. To argue for the welfare of a particular child should not justify practices that will, in the long run, place many children, women, and cultures at risk.

When white and light-skinned Latin or Asian babies are preferred at any price, adoption becomes part of the perpetuation of racism. When women of developing countries are forced into exporting children in increasing numbers for adoption because of rape, poverty, war, political devastation, and the pressure to abandon that results from being located in the world as women with few resources, then adoption perpetuates the practice of robbing women and cultures of children. And when prospective parents go the international adoption route with a studied ignorance and even avoidance of knowing how adoptive children are procured, then intercountry adoption continues as part of the overall reproductive trafficking in women and children.

The United Nations Charter states that intercountry adoption should be a last resort but recognizes the need for it in certain circumstances. Yet when policies and procedures are enacted to safeguard women, children, and cultures from being exploited by adoption trafficking, these same regulations are viewed as obstacles put in the way of Westerners who simply desire to be parents. "Following this logic, prospective adoptive parents are not at fault if they resort to black marketers to help them to acquire their perfect babies fully aware about the questionable channels or fraudulent transactions."[57] In Chile, for one example, where international adoption is not recognized, thousands of children are adopted through illegal channels.

Underlying this demand for children is the patriarchal perception of childlessness as a disease and misfortune that elicits sympathy and pity, a perception that fosters the social pressure not to be childless. As many women endure painful and debilitating reproductive technologies at any cost to themselves, many would-be adoptive parents procure women and their children, at any cost, through the brokering of lawyers, entrepreneurs, and other intermediaries. "Meanwhile we do not only excuse the adoptive parents who encourage such activity but look at them with sympathy. . . . We sympathize with them because we, unfortunately, *still* believe that to be childless is to be a failure."[58]

Surrogate arrangements can only add to this adoption traffic. In the United States, there is evidence that some lawyers who orchestrate private adoptions are now brokering surrogate contracts. For example, the *Cincinnati Enquirer* reported that Katie Brophy, an attorney who arranges surrogate contracts for Richard Levin's Surrogate Parenting Associates of Louisville, Kentucky (the surrogate broker of Elizabeth Kane), has been implicated in controversial private adoption arrangements. Brophy is alleged to have threatened Christine van Wey with the loss of her two daughters after van Wey changed her mind about giving up her son for adoption. Van Wey claimed that she had proceeded with the termination of parental rights agreement only because she had been intimidated and coerced by Brophy. At the same time, Brophy led the adopting parents to believe that she was their lawyer, encouraging them not to hire separate counsel when van Wey initiated legal proceedings to have her child returned.[59]

Adoption, both national and international, must not become a substitute for improving the sex-based conditions of women and their children and for providing material resources for women in need: "From the viewpoint of child welfare policy, . . . priority should not be on adoption but rather on more equitable distribution of income, ensuring universal access to education and health care, the creation of adequate day care programmes and special assistance programmes for families in especially difficult circumstances."[60] Otherwise, intercountry adoption, at best, concentrates a lot of money and assistance on a number of children who are taken away from their mothers, their families, and their countries of origin and, at worst, perpetuates the reproductive trafficking of women and children.

A New Reproductive Traffic: Children for Organ Export?

A new version of the reproductive traffic in women and children is the alleged seizure and sale of children for organ export. Within the last five years, reports of disabled children from Latin America being used for organ extraction have surfaced in the indigenous and international press and have been investigated by human rights organizations. The charges of organ trafficking have been so recurring and extensive that in 1991, the sixteenth session of the UN Working Group on Contemporary Forms of Slavery reviewed all allegations and recommended that all UN groups and institutions such as UNICEF, WHO, and Interpol investigate the allegations further and take action to stop these practices. In a separate hearing at its seventeenth session in 1992, the UN Working Group on Contemporary Forms of Slavery heard testimony on organ trafficking. Verifying the exporting of children for organ use is extremely difficult. The task is like piecing together a giant puzzle in which the pieces do not always fit.

The First Round of Information and Disinformation

One of the first newspaper reports of child organ trafficking came from Central America on January 2, 1987, when *La Tribuna,* a Honduran newspaper, published a story about the baby organ trade out of Honduras. The article quoted the secretary general of the National Council on Social Welfare (JNCS), Leonardo Villeda Bermudez, who maintained that in December 1986 thirteen children were found by Honduran police in four different houses in San Pedro Sula awaiting export to organ providers in the United States. Villeda Bermudez revealed that in these "fattening" houses the children, many of whom were disabled, were being well fed to be "readied" for organ extraction.[61] The French magazine *Jeune Afrique* reported that earlier, in San Pedro Sula, the police had discovered several corpses of children who had already been mutilated and whose organs then went to clandestine private clinics in the United States.[62]

One week later, President Jose Azcona Hoyo denied these allegations of child organ trafficking. The president criticized the remarks of Villeda Bermudez as ill founded, saying that he had based them only on the testimony of one social worker. In an article entitled "¿Ocurrió en el pasado?", translated as "Did It Happen in the Past?", the president was quoted as saying, "They learned that a few adopted children with physical defects *could* have been used."[63] Villeda Bermudez quickly became the ex–secretary general of the National Council of Social Welfare.

In February and March 1987, the Guatemalan newspapers *El Gráfico* and *Prensa Libre* ran a series of articles on a similar organ export scandal in their own country. The articles revealed that the police had discovered a clandestine house in a residential neighborhood in Guatemala City where fourteen newborns, ready for exportation, were found. A national police official, Baudilio Hichos Lopez, stated,

> This trade has existed for a year. There were people who stole the babies, bought them from poor families, or discovered single mothers. They were going to give birth at the clandestine house. In the maternity ward set up there, there was no registration of any of the children born there.

Hichos Lopez also stated that two lawyers, later arrested, negotiated the legal documents to send the children to the United States and added, "We know that these babies are used as organ donors."[64]

Again in March 1987 eight Guatemalans were arrested in three other houses, charged with "kidnapping and illegal trafficking in minors." In one of the houses, eleven children were found, along with ten photocopies of fake birth certificates and nine national identification cards. One of the persons who was detained in this case was Ofelia Rosal de Gama, the sister-in-law of the former military president of Guatemala, Mejía Victores,[65] who was also married to the director of immigration at the time of her detention. The organ trafficking matter was quickly hushed up and witnesses disappeared: "As so often happens in Guatemala nothing more was heard of the case. *Prensa Libre*, noting that people were asking what had happened with the investigation, reported that an Immigration employee who was checking irregularities in passports granted to children being adopted abroad was assassinated on a local city bus."[66]

On April 21, 1987, the Nicaraguan newspaper *Barricada* ran a story about the trafficking of children in Honduras, El Salvador, and Guatemala. This article alleged that in addition to the "fattening houses," private individuals in both official and charitable institutions adopted children with mental or physical handicaps, posing as their benefactors, and then exported them for organ extraction.[67]

A major difficulty in verifying these allegations is that the medical procedure itself would seem to cause many problems in both material and economic terms. When the *International Children's Rights Monitor*, the publication of the Defense for Children International (DCI), consulted medical sources about the organ trafficking reports, questions were raised about the location of the actual operations and the difficulty of concealing the murders or mutilations of the children. Some speculated that the price of such illegally obtained organs would end up being higher than the standard price for organs.[68] And, they asked, how would the organs be preserved for long periods of time? It is, of course, extremely difficult to get specific answers to such questions.

Within the last five years, however, new technologies and drugs have enabled doctors to keep organs for a longer time outside the human body. A new preservation solution, Viaspan, developed by two U.S. scientists and now marketed by Du Pont, ensures that organs can be transported in a preserved state over longer distances and a longer time period. Previously, for example, livers could be kept for only eight hours; with Viaspan, they can be preserved for up to thirty-two hours. And hearts can be preserved for twelve hours instead of the former four-hour time span. If organs can be preserved longer, this obviously answers the question about ability to preserve organs for long distances, thus making it more feasible to traffic organs from one country to another. And like other substances that are part of an illegal and clandestine trafficking network, this preservative could also be obtained by the traffickers.

Nonetheless, as a result of the many unanswered questions regarding the medical issues and the difficulties in obtaining and transporting both the organs and the children, as well as problems in hiding the gruesome evidence, the Defense for Children International took the position that it could not verify the allegations of child organ trafficking. It added, however, that it was "in search of the truth" and that it also found it necessary to publicize summary information on the child organ trafficking reports cited above. Thus, in May 1987 the *International Children's Rights Monitor* (DCI) published a summary of the allegations of child organ trafficking from Central America to European countries and the United States, along with an extremely cautious statement about the allegations.

DCI was immediately reproached by the U.S. Mission to the UN in Geneva. The U.S. Mission pointed out that a Soviet newspaper, *Izvestya,* which had interviewed a DCI staff member, had distorted the DCI representative's remarks, giving them an anti-American bias. For example, *Izvestya* had reported, "There is only one step from American arrogance and racist contempt for the Latin American peoples to total cannibalistic licence." The United States maintained that all subsequent reports of child organ trafficking were based on this Soviet article. It was at this point that the history of child organ trafficking allegations became intertwined with former U.S.-Soviet politics and disinformation.

The United States demanded that DCI issue a denunciation of the article in *Izvestya* and demonstrate how DCI's statements had been manipulated by the Soviets. It added that if DCI failed to make "a clear and unequivocal statement to that effect without delay, the organisation's credibility would be seriously jeopardised . . . and the rumour would be echoed widely in the coming weeks and months in certain media throughout the world."[69]

While DCI agreed that *Izvestya* had indeed distorted its reporting of the interview, it decided initially not to publish a press release. Several months later, rumors began to circulate that DCI was manipulated by the Soviets and that U.S. authorities were questioning the independence of the organization. The Associated Press (U.S.) and Associated Newspapers (U.K.) informed DCI that they were in possession of "damaging information" about DCI's status.

Faced with this international discrediting, DCI finally felt compelled to issue a press release about the *Izvestya* article, stating that it had no information "permitting it either to confirm or deny the rumours relating to the trafficking in organs." While DCI dissociated itself from the ways in which the *Izvestya* article had manipulated some of the DCI representative's remarks, it concluded that it was not easy to say that this was "simply an exercise in disinformation designed to blacken the image of the United States. . . ."[70] DCI also noted that many of the newspapers that published stories in Honduras and Guatemala showed absolutely no anti-U.S. bias. Finally, DCI accused the U.S. representatives of resorting to the same kind of distortions as the Soviets, thereby obfuscating the search for truth.

The Second Round of Information and Disinformation

The allegations of child organ trafficking from Central America to the United States were not to go away. One year later, in 1988, reports again surfaced in the same Guatemalan newspapers (*El Gráfico* and *Prensa Libre*) that seven babies had been rescued who were destined for organ transplants in the United States and Israel. The *El Gráfico* story reported that security agents had captured two Israelis who were working with two Guatemalan lawyers, Jorge Rodolfo Rivera and Carlos Rene Gonzalez, who in turn had enlisted the services of a Guatemalan pediatrician, Joaquin Kackler. They paid women a sum of 50 quetzales (20 dollars) to nurse and care for the babies before they were discovered by personnel of the Narcotics and Intelligence Section (SIN). *El Gráfico* also reported that, according to official information, those captured confessed they had exported children to Israel and the United States so that their organs could be sold for the sum of 75,000 dollars to families who needed transplants for their children.[71]

Three days later, *El Gráfico* published the denial of the Israeli Embassy, which claimed that *El Gráfico* had printed a "monstrous accusation" based on "the irresponsible declarations of a functionary" whose opinion was based on "personal presumptions" and no follow-through investigation. The embassy further declared, "It is impossible to think that in the Land of Israel the aberration and crime of 'butchering children' could be committed." It also stated that organ transplants are prohibited in Israel by law and that "the few cases of transplantations done in Israel were done under very strict conditions of control."[72]

El Gráfico responded to this embassy statement by confirming its story, based on the information it was given by the director of the Intelligence and Narcotics Service (SIN). It made clear that it was not singling out the State of Israel or the United States for these abuses, nor was it saying that it was the policy of these countries to allow such outrages to occur.

However, the U.S. Embassy in Guatemala claimed that *El Gráfico* printed a "clarification" two days after it broke the original report. This "clarification" supposedly stated that the newspaper no longer believed the government functionary's statement. In a phone interview with the Guatemalan Health Rights Project, however, *El Gráfico* stated that the paper stood by its original story and had not printed any retraction or apology.[73] Dr. Carlos Soto, the minister of health, replied to all inquiries about the story with a terse three liner declaring that the initial *El Gráfico* article was untrue. He mentioned nothing about later articles alleging the exporting of children and organs.

In 1988 newspaper accounts from Peru detailed the story of Rosita, whose eyes were seized by organ traffickers before Rosita's mother could take her away from the house in which she worked. According to Dr. Carmen Meza Ingar, president of the Peruvian Association of Women Lawyers, organ dealers usually kill their victims, so it is fortunate that Rosita and her mother ultimately escaped. The Peruvian police are trying to locate Rosita and her mother to provide testimony to the court of justice about the alleged eye snatching. At the same time, the Peruvian Police (PIP) homicide section, together with the Supreme Penal Attorney, carried out surprise inspections of medical centers suspected of being linked to the organ trafficking "mafia." Dr. Carmen Meza Ingar also stated that this "mafia" of organ dealers supplies research and transplantation centers in Europe and Japan. In 1988 the organ mafia reportedly began operating out of Peru because its agents had been arrested in Venezuela, Colombia, Argentina, and Honduras, where they had been from 1986 to 1988.[74]

In November 1988 the European Parliament in Belgium passed a resolution condemning the trafficking in children from Central America and the sale of children for organ transplants. The resolution was initiated by a French Communist member, Danielle de March. The European Parliament's strong condemnation of the reported organ trafficking is substantively different from most governmental responses to allegations of organ trafficking, which typically take one of two forms. As with sexual trafficking, governments most often report there is no problem. Obviously, such trafficking is illegal and would reflect badly on the image of a country; therefore it does not exist. Newspapers that report abuses in this area are accused of sensationalism and disinformation and of not being able to verify their stories. Or they have been accused of communist sympathies and of being dominated by "foreign-supported radical Marxists." This was the conventional response of the United States to the baby organ trade allegations in 1987.

In the summer of 1988, U.S. Information Agency (USIA) officials tried to halt what they termed "a rash of unsubstantiated reports in the world press that Latin American slum children are being sold to provide organ transplants for wealthy U.S. buyers."[75] First reported in the *Washington Post*, the story was subheadlined: "U.S. Combats Soviet-Fostered Reports of Latin Youngsters Sold to Provide Organ Transplants." Labeling the durability of such reports as partly due to the Soviet Union's "disinformation propaganda apparatus," Herbert Romerstein, chief advisor on disinformation activities to USIA, constructed an extensive chronology of events relating to the sale of children for organ extraction based on what he said were Soviet efforts to spread such a history. This chronology was sent to U.S. embassies and consulates throughout the world as a tool in refuting the organ export allegations.

In summary, Romerstein's chronology is based on the following refutations. All charges of organ trafficking in both 1987 and 1988, Romerstein contends, can be traced back to a story in the Honduran newspaper, *La Tribuna*, in which a senior government official, Leonardo Villeda Bermudez, was quoted (see above). Romerstein maintains that Villeda Bermudez immediately repudiated the story of organized trafficking in babies for body parts and also that he had made no charges but had only casually mentioned "unconfirmed rumors."[76] Romerstein does not mention that Villeda Bermudez lost his position as secretary general of the National Council of Social Welfare one week after these allegations were made. Nor does it mention that he may have repudiated such allegations because he was forced to in the wake of the denial of the president of Honduras, who said that such organ trafficking could never happen in Honduras.

In the *Washington Post* article, Romerstein contends that the Honduran story then spread to Guatemalan newspapers, *not* that officials in Guatemala discovered independent organ trafficking occurring in their own country. When I interviewed John Goshko, who wrote the "disinformation" story for the *Washington Post,* I mentioned that the newspaper *El Gráfico,* which originally broke the story in Guatemala, was published by Jorge Carpio Nicolle, a right-wing presidential candidate, who recently ran again in the Guatemalan presidential elections. How then, I asked, could *El Gráfico*'s story be construed as communist inspired? Goshko responded that no matter what political party one belonged to, there was a "confluence of anti-American opinion in Central America." He added that he "would take these newspaper reports with a grain of salt, because the Central American press is very unreliable."[77]

Continuing with the chronology, Romerstein stated that the Honduran story supposedly was then circulated in other news media, escalating the rumors in other parts of Central America and the Caribbean. *Pravda* entered the picture on April 5, 1987, when it published a dispatch from its Mexico City correspondent—one that repeated the original Honduran allegations of Villeda Bermudez but omitted his subsequent disclaimers.[78] Romerstein noted that in subsequent months, the story was picked up by other communist-controlled newspapers such as *Barricada* in Nicaragua and *L'Humanité* in France but sometimes too in mainstream newspapers.

In the wake of prompt and official governmental denials in Honduras, Guatemala, the United States, and Israel, the story died down until it was resurrected in August 1987 by a Reuters news dispatch in which a Brazilian judge alleged organ trafficking from Brazil to Paraguay. The dispatch, carried by many Western papers, reported that babies had been kidnapped in Brazil and then transported to Paraguay destined for organ banks in the United States. It based this report on the testimony of Judge Angel Campos, who at that time presided over the juvenile court in Asunción and who found that seven Brazilian baby boys were rescued from a Paraguayan transit house, along with five Brazilian women who were arrested on charges of kidnapping.[79]

The kidnappers apparently pretended that the babies—from six months to three years old—were going to be adopted in the United States. Suspicions arose, the judge said, when the court was told that the supposed parents wanted any type of baby, even those who were "deformed." Most adoptive parents, he said, request healthy and pretty children.

In chronicling and commenting on the Reuters story, the *Washington Post* said "The judge's remarks later proved to be unsubstantiated variations on the story that originated in Honduras,"[80] a claim that is difficult to square with the fact that the judge protested a quite independent case of seven Brazilian children destined for organ transplants. Indeed, what Romerstein and the *Washington Post* claim is all of a piece in Honduras, Guatemala, and Paraguay is hardly the same story. However, at the prompting of upset U.S. officials, Reuters ran another article reinforcing the "seamless garment" version of the child organ trafficking "rumors" and saying that the judge's allegations were unsubstantiated. In the meantime, the first Reuters dispatch had traveled far and wide and was published in many Western countries. At this point, Romerstein claims that the International Association of Democratic Lawyers (IADL)—what he refers to as a Soviet surrogate in Brussels—submitted a long unsubstantiated report to the UN Human Rights subcommission in Geneva recycling the same version of disinformation about the child organ trafficking. When the European Parliament passed its resolution in November 1988 the U.S. State Department criticized it for basing the resolution on "false and misleading statements and a discredited report by a Soviet front organization." The State Department also noted that the resolution was introduced by a French Communist and was approved without debate. It added that "the U.S. government has made an exhaustive investigation and concluded the charges are 'totally groundless.'"[81]

Throughout 1987 and 1988 U.S. governmental officials continued to deny that babies and/or organs had been exported to the United States from Central America. They charged that the facts were unsubstantiated and that allegations were no more than rumors and communist-inspired disinformation. Yet the rumors have stubbornly persisted through two rounds of trying to kill off such supposed disinformation. Why, for example, has there been no serious investigation of these 1987 and 1988 charges in Guatemala? It is well established that countless numbers of children have been taken out of Central American countries for adoption in the United States and Europe, often illegally. As the Nicaraguan newspaper *Barricada* noted, the sudden rise in the price of children for export from 3,000 dollars previously to the current price of 10,000 dollars fuels the speculation that "traffickers in children have discovered an activity even more lucrative than adoption."[82]

Despite all previous attempts by the U.S. government to treat the allegations of organ trafficking as simply the result of a prior Soviet-based disinformation campaign, another serious charge of organ trafficking from Brazil to Italy surfaced in 1990. In September of that year, both the *Guardian* in London and *la Repubblica* in Italy reported the existence of an Italian criminal organization that allegedly operated an organ network.[83] Italian authorities reportedly asked Interpol to investigate charges that the Napolitan *camorra*, a highly organized criminal group, is transporting disabled children to Italy and then passing them on to other countries for illicit organ transplants. *La Repubblica* also reported that Italian magistrates have confirmed that over four thousand children, most of them from Brazil, have been sent to Italy since 1986. Yet only one thousand children have been verifiably adopted by Italians during this period. Children come into the country with adoption visas, yet most adoptions are not then regularized in the Italian courts. It is possible that Italy serves as a transitional location for children who move on to other countries for adoption, but this does not account for the large numbers. Thus three thousand children may have become part of a criminally run international organ market with transplants taking place not only in suspected countries such as Thailand and Mexico, but also in European clinics.

The *camorra* is alleged to be behind the organ trafficking. Many Italian couples who have brought South American children into the country reside in areas of the Italian state of Campania where the *camorra* rules. A second implicating factor involves the couples' requests for medical certificates documenting children's blood groups and subgroups and data on particular organs. Finally, Brazil has also been a refuge of many *camorrists* wanted by the Italian police.

Other circumstances establish a Brazil-Italy connection. The British *Guardian* reported that an Italian expriest turned lawyer, Lucas di Nuzzo, admitted that he procured Brazilian children for many Italians by channeling them through a refuge that he ran for homeless and orphaned children and by finding Brazilian couples to act as false parents who would then sign documents releasing them for adoption. In addition, some Brazilian mothers testified that their children had disappeared and were taken without their consent. In other places in Brazil, vans that drive around remote areas collecting children for vaccinations have been implicated in these disappearances. Police have also found houses in which babies, usually bought from poor illiterate women, were kept. Alleged participants in this organ network have been arrested by Brazilian police but later released on bail while awaiting trial, which in Brazil can take years.[84]

In 1991, when Latin America's Roman Catholic bishops met in Buenos Aires, Argentina, they condemned the "killing of Latin American children," who they say in some cases are "committed for the sale of body parts to First World countries."[85] Peruvian bishop Luis Amrando Barbaren Gastelumendi of Chimbote told the Catholic News Service that there is a small but growing movement to "eliminate poor or physically limited" children for the sale of body parts in Peru, and that his comments on the organ trade have led the Peruvian government to form a commission to investigate the matter.[86]

Finally in April 1992 both the *British Medical Journal* and *The Lancet* carried articles on alleged murders of patients killed for their organs at a state-run psychiatric institute in Argentina. Testimonies from health workers at the Montes de Oca Mental Health Institute in Lujan led Argentine judicial officials to exhume the bodies of former patients of the institute whose corneas and other organs were found missing. "Government investigators claim that corneas and other organs were sold by Dr. Sanchez and his accomplices and that patients' blood was drained for storage in the blood bank of his own private clinic."[87] Authorities are trying to establish whether the organs were sold abroad through networks of organ dealers who are part of an international traffic in organs and body parts. Health workers state that the allegations are not new and that during the past three or four years, reports of missing children have surfaced from time to time. Furthermore, two years ago, a member of the institute staff, Dr. A. Jubileo, disappeared, and her body has not been found. "It was seriously presumed then that she had been eliminated because she had found out about the goings-on at the institute."[88] Since there is no independent oversight mechanism to investigate irregularities in the health care sector in Argentina, those working within the state health system are not surprised and expect that few results will be forthcoming from these discoveries and any subsequent investigation. Complicating any investigation is the way in which the government has created past scandals to draw attention away from corruption by the president's relatives and friends.[89]

Behind the Organ Trafficking Allegations: Myth or Reality?

Allegations of organ trafficking have been largely attributed to past Soviet disinformation campaigns but, increasingly, other rationalizations are offered to discount the charges. Some academic explanations take the form of a kind of "middle knowledge—something one knows and does not know . . . a combination of knowledge and numbing, but the knowledge seeps through."[90] For example, in a paper presented at a symposium of the American Ethnological Society in April 1990 entitled "Bodies, Death, and the State: Violence and the Taken-for-Granted World," anthropologist Nancy Scheper-Hughes discusses the organ-snatching beliefs of Brazilian shantytown residents as an example of "mundane surrealism." She views their fears as a blending of fiction and fact that creates a kind of mass hysteria about "what could possibly happen . . . [a] collective delirium . . . [in which] rumors of organ and body snatching have their basis in poor people's everyday encounters with a modern biotechnomedical reality that does, in fact, view and treat their bodies and body parts as 'dispensable.'"[91] However, the reality is that in Brazil, the lives of the poor are cheap, children are abandoned and do disappear, poor people's experiences with clinics and hospitals do leave their bodies damaged and mutilated, many do not return from hospitals, and an anxiety develops about what could happen. In this context, it makes more sense to view the organ seizure fears and rumors, *not as separate* from the overall situation, but as one more part of the very material circumstances of children's disappearances and medical mutilations.

Another example of a "middle-knowledge" explanation appeared in the U.S. feminist newspaper *New Directions for Women*. Entitled "'Baby Parts' Myth Explained," author Louise Palmer discounts the organ

trafficking allegations in South and Central America as myth. Treating
South America as a "breeding ground for myths," Palmer attributes the
persistence of the organ trafficking rumors to several things. In these
countries, she cites "a dislike and distrust of foreigners entrenched in
the national psyches" but especially aimed at North Americans, who have
exercised an economic and cultural hegemony over their South American neighbors for years and exploited their people and resources. Other
factors are the infant mortality rates in some Latin American countries,
which have doubled over the last decade, as well as the number of children living in utter poverty. Poverty has been exacerbated by a massive
foreign debt, which has helped slash social services, force abandonment
of children, and create a booming market in illicit adoptions fueled by
North American demand. The author quotes a Mexican adoption specialist, Victor Carlos Garcia, who states that the widespread acceptance
of the baby parts stories is linked to this adoption market.

> Children are being bought, sold and "exported," although not for
> their organs.
> The "baby-parts" story, unlike its subject, seems destined to have a
> long shelf-life. Although the story may have no basis in fact, it points
> to a very real legacy of exploitation that the Third World has yet to
> escape. Until it does, such stories will appear, offering the same meta-
> phor, the same characters, the same circumstances.[92]

In this explanation, the rumors of baby organ trafficking testify to
the inability of South and Central American societies who are often not
able to sustain their children. However, there is no reason for adoptions
to be pitted against organ trafficking, using the former to discount the
latter. It is clear from an extensive examination of adoption trafficking
patterns that these same routes could be used for organ trafficking and,
if anything, have paved the way for the organ trade. Moreover, the same
individuals and groups that have advertised babies for adoption appear
now to be selling human organs for transplantation. In 1988, the *British
Medical Journal* reported that Count Adelmann of Karlsruhe, well
known in Germany for offering South American babies for adoption,
advertised human kidneys for transplantation by French surgeons in
Paris.[93]

Social critic Noam Chomsky offers a similar conclusion in a two-part critical article on the U.S. "victory" for democracy in Eastern Europe, Latin and South America, and elsewhere. In this article, entitled "The Victors: I and II," Chomsky relates how the U.S.-imposed development model has emphasized "nontraditional exports" from South and Central American countries in recent years. In part 1 of this article, he summarizes the reports of organ trafficking emanating from Honduras, Guatemala, and El Salavador, cautiously affirming their validity. At the same time, he states that the reports could not be confirmed by the International Human Rights Federation but that they were widely believed in the region. In part 2, however, Chomsky summarily dismisses these same allegations in Brazil. "Here too it is widely alleged that babies are sacrificed for organ banks, a belief that can hardly be true but that reveals much about the conditions under which it takes root."[94] Like the *New Directions* article, Chomsky implies that homeless and starving children, death squads who kill abandoned and poor children in the streets of Brazil, and the general contempt in which the lives of the poor are held create the conditions in which these allegations—not these realities—flourish.

Chomsky, Palmer, and Scheper-Hughes use conditions of exploitation, poverty, and general cheapness of the lives of the underclass in South and Central American countries to dimiss the organ trade. Their tendency to see organ snatching as *separate from rather than as integral to* the widespread conditions of exploitation in South and Central America is unfortunate. From all the material presented thus far, it makes just as much sense to view allegations of organ trafficking as very much related to these factors: the widespread sexual and reproductive exploitation of women and children; the extensive traffic in adoption that is acknowledged by all governments in Latin America and by many in the West; the ravaging of indigenous resources and the culture of abject poverty; the disappearances and medical mutilations of children that occur every day; and the abandonment of children. These conditions confirm the need to view child organ trafficking not as distinct from but as part of the overall organized structure of the varied sexual and reproductive trafficking in women and children worldwide. In addition, Chomsky, Palmer, and Scheper-Hughes have not examined the allegations of organ trafficking in a systematic and serious way but merely speculate from one set of conditions to another.

Let me summarize the evidence for organ trafficking and distill conclusions from the allegations that have been documented thus far in this chapter. Indigenous government officials who initially reported organ trafficking either disappear or are demoted. For example, in the aftermath of revealing the existence of "fattening houses" in Honduras, Villeda Bermudez, secretary general of the National Council of Social Welfare, quickly left his post. Immigration authorities, who have discovered irregularities in children's passports as they exit from the country, have been assassinated in Guatemala. In addition, individuals who have been implicated in organ trafficking and who have high governmental connections, such as Rosal de Gama in Guatemala, have not been investigated or prosecuted, and then public protests are muted.

Not only have individuals been silenced or "disappeared," but also strong-arm tactics have been used to repress international human rights groups, such as the Defense for Children International (DCI), that have issued even very cautious statements about the organ trafficking allegations or that simply call for an investigation. Most indigenous and Western governments have not conducted any serious investigations into the charges, some have summarily denied the existence of an organ trade from or to their respective countries, and others such as Guatemala have issued contradictory statements saying that the traffic was not happening in their country while at the same time saying it "couldn't happen if the adoption laws were stricter."

In spite of these silencing strategies, many governmental and nongovernmental groups have not been intimidated and have taken the allegations seriously enough to issue resolutions and call for full-scale investigations of organ trafficking. In 1988 the European Parliament issued a resolution condemning the trafficking and sale of children for organs from Central America (see above). In the same year, Regula Bott, a progressive member of the West German Bundestag, submitted a petition of forty-two questions to the German Parliament calling for an intensive investigation into the "Organhandel" and "Kinderhandel" (organ and children trafficking) from the Third World to Germany.[95] Three years later, the Latin American bishops council, CELAM, condemned the kidnapping, illegal adoption, and killing of Latin American children for body parts. And in August 1991 the UN Economic and Social Council's Working Group on Contemporary Forms of Slavery reviewed allegations of the organ trafficking and alerted other UN groups such as WHO and Interpol to investigate and take action.

Western governments continue to claim that the child organ allegations were the result of a Soviet-inspired disinformation campaign, especially against the United States. However, in the midst of this supposed Soviet conspiracy, it is important to recall that some of the indigenous newspapers that reported the stories of child organ exports, such as *El Gráfico* in Guatemala, were notoriously anticommunist. Additionally, these charges have persisted in the aftermath of the cold war, as seen in the 1990 allegations of child organ trafficking between Brazil and Italy. And in Argentina the bodies of psychiatric patients, which had been raided for organs, were found, although we do not yet know whether these organs were trafficked internationally.

Groups such as the *camorra* link the country of organ origin with the country of organ destination, strongly implicating organized criminal groups in the organ trafficking. For example, after seeking refuge in Brazil from criminal prosecution in Italy, the *camorra* is suspected of transporting children from Brazil back to Italy, where the children are then adopted or passed on to organ suppliers.

Finally, the number of countries in South and Central America where these allegations have surfaced—Honduras, Guatemala, El Salvador, Peru, Brazil, Mexico, Paraguay, and Colombia—testifies to the independence, not the dependence, of these charges from country to country. The U.S. Information Agency (USIA), for example, constructed an elaborate chronology making organ trafficking allegations in one country dependent on similar allegations in a prior country. The multiplicity of countries where allegations surfaced was thus explained by a contagiousness of rumor-mongering in which each country's allegations were linked to prior allegations in Central and South America. But this contagiousness theory is called into question by the persistence of quite independent discoveries of organ trafficking in quite different countries. Moreover, the contagiousness theory, or the supposition that these allegations are all of the same cloth, masks the recognition of the *real network* of organ traffickers who may be connected throughout Central and South America and who indeed are connected with each other. For example, findings from the Peruvian Association of Women Lawyers link the existence of the organ mafia in Peru to their being driven out of other countries in Central and South America.

The sexual, reproductive, and drug trafficking that is proven to exist provides already-established routes and contacts for organs to be transported. The sudden rise in the cost of international adoptions, the many children bound for adoption in countries such as Italy who were never regularized through national legal adoption channels, and the entrance of known adoption brokers, like Count Adelmann of Germany, into the organ business is powerful circumstantial evidence for the existence of international organ trafficking.

Given the demand for organs in the United States, it is also plausible that the organ supply would be coming from somewhere relatively near. The demand for organ transplants has increased sharply in the North, where thousands of expectant organ recipients die each year. Even if voluntary donations increased from the families of dying patients, this would not provide for all the organ requests, which continue to grow rapidly. The supply has remained at about four thousand donors for the past four years.[96] However, the United Network for Organ Sharing (UNOS) documented that in 1989, 17,578 people were waiting for organ transplants. UNOS also publishes a numerical breakdown of people waiting for kidney, heart, liver, lung, pancreas, and heart-lung transplants.

There is much controversy regarding the best method of obtaining consent for organ donation. The United Kingdom uses an "opt-in" system requiring the signing of a donor card and relatives' consent. But some believe that this system fails to meet the need for organs and is outmoded and should be changed to an "opt-out" system in which it is assumed that people want to donate their organ unless they have registered a prior objection to donation. This system currently operates in Austria, Belgium, and France.

Complicating any system of organ donation is what happens to the bodies of deceased once they go to postmortem. In Australia, for example, Dr. Lynette Dumble, senior research fellow in transplant surgery at the University of Melbourne, argues that the 1982 Human Tissue Act of Victoria is so loose that organs can be harvested from the dead without family permission on the grounds that they have therapeutic value.

In this way, she contends, pituitary glands were harvested from human brains in the 1980s to manufacture growth and fertility hormones.[97] If organ raiding takes place so easily, and effectively illegally, in Western hospital mortuaries, these actions lend support to the ability of organ traffickers to harvest organs in less restricted contexts.

In the wake of these controversies, many reputable physicians and businessmen have called for compensation for donors or their families and for paying live donors. In 1990 *Forbes* magazine, one of the largest business magazines in the United States, ran a story advocating that people be allowed to buy and sell organs. The author cited the example of poorer countries, where buying organs from living donors in a straightforward commercial transaction has become the only real solution for patients with kidney failure. The saying among transplant specialists in India, for example, is, "Either I buy, or they die." "Thus are organs literally human capital."[98]

Currently, however, the U.S. National Organ Transplant Act of 1984 makes the buying and selling of organs an illegal act punishable by fines of up to 50,000 dollars, five years in prison, or both. Furthermore, in 1985 the World Medical Association proposed legislation against organ trading in all countries, but not every country observes the ban.[99] Given the demand for organs that has been documented above, however, it is possible that those who are desperate for organs may be turning to a Central and South American organ trade that has been allegedly in operation for at least five years. Also, organ brokers may well be taking advantage of the momentum for the commercialization of organs, establishing currently illegal routes of export in preparation for the day when organ exports will be legalized. At that point, they may be ready to move into the legal commerce.

As we have seen, critics have questioned the supply from developing countries as myth or as the exaggerations of conditions of poverty, the adoption trade, and medical crimes that exist in nations where organ trafficking is said to flourish. Few have addressed the demand factor and the pressure for organs from those in need. However, the large demand for organs raises the questions of where these organs will come from and, indeed, where they are now coming from. The issue of demand leads us to examine the trafficking in fetal tissue.

The Trafficking in Fetal Parts and Tissue

Early reports about the trafficking in human organs also addressed a trade in fetal organs and tissue. In 1988 *Jeune Afrique* published allegations about a long-standing involvement of the U.S. government in buying fetal parts from Korea. The article summarized international press accounts, beginning with the 1976 revelations of *Asahi Shimbun*, the largest Japanese daily newspaper. *Asahi Shimbun* reported that more than twenty thousand fetal kidneys were imported to the United States from South Korea for military research. The article, in turn, quoted M. Lee Myong Bok, a professor at the University of Seoul, who acknowledged that he performed cesarian sections on women who were up to eight months pregnant, "under pretext of complications."[100] He stated that until 1969 Flow Laboratories, a Rockville, Maryland, pharmaceutical company, paid him 15 dollars for a pair of fetal kidneys, a cost that gradually increased to 30 dollars. At that time, Flow was the number one provider of human tissue in the world.[101]

The *Jeune Afrique* article also referred to a 1986 *Washington Post* article alleging that between 1970 and 1976 laboratories of the U.S. Department of Defense had imported from South Korea twelve thousand pairs of kidneys taken from three- to eight-month-old fetuses. During these years, there would have been a large supply of fetuses for export, since by 1970 the number of abortions in South Korea approximated its birth rate and eight years later induced abortions were three times the number of births.[102]

French author Roland Girard, in a book on the trade in human organs, specifically cited a U.S. medical military research laboratory at Fort Detrick, Maryland, which bought fetal tissue cultures for research on infectious diseases. Between 1970 and 1980, Girard reported that about eighty thousand seven- to eight-month-old fetuses had been imported annually to the United States from around the world.[103] He wrote that during a television interview on French TV (TFI), the U.S. undersecretary of state admitted that the importing of fetal organs from South Korea to U.S. medical military labs was in existence until 1977. The undersecretary cautioned, however, that this tissue was only used for attempts at isolating naturally occurring diseases. After the publicity that was generated over the exporting of fetal organs to the United States, South Korea ceased its controversial exports.[104]

In 1985 a West German Social Democrat testified before the Council of Europe alleging the existence of an international trade in embryos for "commercial purposes." He stated that in March 1981 French customs officials seized a consignment of embryos from Romania, on their way to a California manufacturer of beauty products. In 1982 the California police seized another five hundred embryos intended for cosmetics production. The politician, Horst Haase, asked the Parliamentary Assembly of the Council of Europe for legislation banning commercial and industrial uses of embryos, in keeping with its declarations and directives on human rights. Nevertheless, Haase contends that the legislation stalled in committee because lobbyists for scientists and the pharmaceutical industry inhibited any passage of such legislation.[105]

In 1985 the *Daily Mail* in London and the BBC reported that British companies were involved in the trading of aborted fetuses for similar commercial purposes. Australian newspaper reports also alleged that fetuses, as well as organs from fetuses, were offered for sale and bought by laboratories to develop cosmetics.[106] The trafficking and the use of fetal organs and tissue for commercial products have been eclipsed by the recent medical pleas for fetal tissue in the research and treatment of diseases such as Huntington's and Alzheimer's.

Medical research involving fetal tissue has been going on for decades, but only recently has it been used in actually treating patients. Thus it has been difficult to raise objections, since challenging the use of fetal tissue is portrayed as opposing medical treatment that not only could benefit a large number of people but could cure the worst kind of diseases from which people suffer.

Fetal Tissue as the New Medical Miracle

Fetal tissue is widely used in medical experiments because it grows rapidly and easily in laboratory conditions and resembles cancer cells, thus enabling scientists to investigate what controls cell growth. Medical researchers have speculated that such tissue will be particularly useful in treating diseases of degenerative cell destruction. Fetal organs, used in transplantation, also adapt well, developing until they take over the failing organ and posing less threat of rejection. Indeed, fetal cells seem filled with scientific promise. Yet no one really knows whether fetal cells can live up to that promise.

Like other scientific discoveries discussed in this book, fetal tissue has been publicized as a miracle cure for all sorts of neurological diseases in which grafts of fetal brain tissue are expected to divide and grow, thus producing neural cells to replace the diseased ones. However, future proposals go beyond the treatment of neurological diseases and injuries to use of fetal pancreases for diabetes mellitus or fetal livers for certain blood and metabolic disorders. Fetal liver cells have been used already in the treatment of radiation-induced bone marrow failure and could be used for other bone marrow diseases, such as leukemia and aplastic anemia, and for certain blood and clotting disorders, such as hemophilia. Embryonic and early fetal cells might also be employed in various forms of genetic therapy. However, the claims that are now being made for the promising use of fetal tissue are just that—claims. In the area of fetal tissue research, we have eschatological medicine married to an eagerly adoring media at its finest—more promise than performance.

Author Peter McCullagh, in reviewing much of the medical literature on fetal transplantation and on fetal tissue's supposed immunological benefits, demonstrates that the original and primary studies on fetal transplantation provide little or no reliable data. McCullagh stresses that many are badly flawed or selectively documented as well as based on second-hand misreporting by scientific specialists.[107]

Operations using fetal tissue took place first in Mexico City and then in Stockholm, Sweden, and Birmingham, England. The University of Colorado joined the medical fray, performing the first U.S. fetal tissue transplant in November 1988. Because the number of surgeries performed remains relatively small, however, information about the results of fetal transplant operations is sparse. Still, popular articles in Western countries, including Britain and the United States, continue to insist that fetal tissue is a miracle cure, especially for Parkinson's disease. Asked by Ted Koppel on ABC's "Nightline" if fetal tissue will cure

people of Parkinson's, Dr. Rene Drucker Colin, head of the Department
of Neuroscience at the National University of Mexico, replied,

> No, it's not a cure. It's a procedure which improves the patient's
> symptoms. The cure, since we don't know what causes Parkinson's dis-
> ease, obviously you can't cure it. It's a degenerative disease and the
> cells that are damaged are still damaged.[108]

Furthermore, what little we know about the actual results of the
surgeries done thus far are cause for caution, not a case for cure. The
first reported example of grafting tissue from the brain of a spontane-
ously aborted human fetus to a Parkinson's patient happened in Mexico
City in 1987. Only eight weeks after the operation, Ignacio Madrazo and
his colleagues from the La Raza Medical Center claimed "an evident
objective improvement in the symptoms of Parkinson's disease." The
claim was made in a letter to the January 1988 *New England Journal of
Medicine* but provided few details of the procedure. *Science News*
reported that many scientists "express skepticism about those results,
with some scientists' questions verging upon accusations of exaggeration."[109] A year earlier, the Mexicans claimed to dramatically improve
the condition of several Parkinson's patients with grafts of adrenal
medulla from the patients' own bodies. Yet three of the eight Mexican
patients had died within two years of the operation, probably as a result
of it.[110]

After the Mexican operation, Anders Bjorklund and colleagues in
Sweden reported in 1988 that they had performed two fetal grafts on
patients with Parkinson's disease. The actual grafts were done at the end
of 1987, but the Swedes delayed reporting the operations to protect the
patients and to evaluate the results over a longer period than the Mexican team. Many neurologists had waited for the Swedish results before
deciding whether to perform fetal transplant surgery themselves, but
what they heard was not encouraging. Olle Lindvall, the neurologist on
the team, announced that there had been "no therapeutic improvement" from the procedure.[111] The two women patients who had undergone fetal tissue transplants from the brains of human fetuses were
producing no more dopamine in their brains after the operation than
before. Another member of the Swedish team admitted, "The results

have not been impressive. The implantations . . . have not had any clinical significance."[112]

As basic assumptions about fetal tissue transplants were called into question, some investigators asked about the wisdom of pursuing more widespread surgery on humans. Donald Gash, a pioneer in brain cell transplants said, "This is still a procedure that has a high morbidity, a high mortality, and patients that have Parkinson's disease do have access to good treatment by conventional means with which they can live a normal life span." Other scientists stated that there is no clear evidence that cell grafts are really surviving in humans and no way of ruling out factors not related to the grafts that contribute to patients' recovery.[113]

The Swedish results, in particular, caused the American Academy of Neurology (AAN) to issue a position statement on the use of fetal tissue transplantation in the treatment of Parkinson's disease. "We urge great caution in expanding the current human experience except as research conducted in highly specialized centers."[114] Responding to the unseemly haste with which many clinical centers were embarking on fetal tissue surgery, the AAN recommended further transplant studies on animals.

Two weeks earlier, the American Association of Neurological Surgeons, at their annual meeting, had issued warnings about performing fetal tissue surgery. This admonition was issued in spite of a report from a University of Colorado team stating that the first patient in the United States to receive a graft of fetal tissue was demonstrating substantial improvement six months after surgery.[115]

Despite the reservations expressed by the professional groups of neurosurgeons and neurologists, fetal cells remain the tissue of choice for neuroscientists. Researchers continue to perform experimental transplants of fetal tissue into the brains of Parkinson's patients in the wake of largely discouraging results. And people who have no other hope are lining up to be recipients for fetal tissue grafts that may do them no good and may even do them harm. As one commentator in the *New Scientist* wrote, "A more difficult question concerns why some doctors are engaging in what is clearly an experimental procedure on the basis of rather limited scientific evidence of its efficacy. . . . It is hard to have to admit that while other branches of medicine have some claim to offering cures for their patients, neurology is comparatively empty-handed."[116] In 1990 a report prepared for UNESCO, "Human Rights Aspects of Transactions in Body Parts and Human Fetuses," found that "the available reports [on fetal tissue transplantation] emphasize progress rather than problems" and that despite great initial enthusiasm, "its promise has not been fulfilled."[117]

Nevertheless, newspaper headlines in November 1992 once more reported clinical success using fetal tissue to repair the brains of a small group of Parkinson's patients. The text of the article, however, told a different story. The *Boston Globe*, for example, reported that the technique "did not alleviate all symptoms or achieve consistent results." Three patients gained "modest improvement," and one patient died four months after the implant surgery. The results of eight other patients "could not be discussed." Success, it seems, was limited to two persons who were not suffering from Parkinson's but had become literally frozen in place after injecting themselves with a tainted synthetic heroin. They were depicted as regaining the ability to walk, dress, feed, and groom themselves. Researchers also admitted that to improve the survival rate of transplanted tissue, multiple abortions would have to be scheduled within hours of the fetal implant operation because only 10 percent of the implanted fetal cells survive. Clearly this latter issue raises questions about the even larger amount of fetal tissue that is needed and where it will come from.

The Facts, Figures, and Methods of Obtaining Fetal Tissue

Like adoption and organ trafficking, the world of fetal tissue procurement is very murky. There are no good figures on the number of fetuses used in medical research, but there are indications that it is substantial. To meet this demand, suppliers in the United States may procure a certain amount of tissue from abroad, as happened in the 1960s and 1970s for military research. It is reported that 90 percent of researchers get fetal tissue through private arrangements with fetal tissue processing companies, abortion clinics, or gynecologists.[118]

Currently, the largest U.S. supplier of fetal tissue is the Institute for the Advancement of Medicine, a nonprofit company in Effington, Pennsylvania. The institute pays rental fees of 500 to 1,000 dollars a month to abortion clinics, depending on whether institute employees spend several days or an entire week processing fetal tissue there.[119] Other suppliers of fetal tissue reimburse clinics for each tissue sample. Although some federal and state regulations forbid paying women for fetal tissue from abortions, procurement agencies can reimburse abortion clinics 25 to 50 dollars per fetal tissue sample. Currently, clinics have to pay for disposing of tissue, and reimbursement gives them a financial incentive to hand over fetal tissue to suppliers.

Hana Biologics, a California-based company specializing in fetal cell research and distribution, estimates that the potential market in treating diabetes and Parkinson's disease through the use of fetal tissue from induced abortion exceeds 6 billion dollars. Stewart Newman of the New York Medical College says, "As various interest groups become accustomed to and dependent upon supplies of fetal tissue they will inevitably seek to enforce their rights to this material."[120] Thus a vast and lucrative market could be created for the tissue.

In 1988 the Institute for the Advancement of Medicine insisted that its clinic and hospital suppliers obtain a woman's consent before giving over the fetal tissue. About half of the suppliers refused and no longer provide the institute with tissue, indicating the perception that a substantial number of women if asked would refuse. However, even if all women undergoing elective abortions consented to their fetal tissue being used for medical research, there would still not be enough to meet the demand.

At the present time 1.5 million elective abortions are performed yearly in the United States, about 80 percent of which are done in the first trimester. Of these first trimester abortions, 94 percent are performed by the suction and curettage method in which most of the fetal matter is rendered unusable for medical purposes. Particularly where fetal brain cells are being transplanted, it is difficult to identify brain tissue after it is macerated by suction and curettage. In the aftermath of such abortion methods, it has been estimated that only 10 percent of fetal tissue is usable. Thus, in principle, approximately 90,000 early fetuses could be available for transplantation use each year.[121]

The annual incidence of Parkinson's disease in the United States is approximately 60,000 new cases per year. However, Parkinson's is not the only disease for which fetal tissue is proposed. At the present time 2.5 million people suffer from Alzheimer's disease, 15,000 people are diagnosed each year as insulin-dependent diabetics, 300,000 are victims of spinal cord or neural tissue injuries, and more than 10,000 individuals suffer from hemophilia, muscular dystrophy, and Huntington's disease. The list of proposed uses for fetal tissue is endless and thus, the proposed medical research and experimentation for fetal tissue is unlimited.

Seldom noted in discussions about the ethics of fetal tissue procurement are how the methods of abortion must be altered to obtain intact fetal tissue. To get usable tissue during the first trimester of pregnancy, the Institute for the Advancement of Medicine encourages doctors to employ ultrasound to find the fetus in the woman's uterus and then to use the suction method, varying the amount of suction to try and trap the whole fetus in the catheter. However, this method is not hugely successful. One doctor who procured tissue for the institute said that he had developed a suction technique that allowed him to extract intact first trimester fetuses 80 percent of the time. Abortions using this method take fifteen to twenty-five minutes instead of the usual five to seven minutes.[122] Australian doctors admit that the preferred method of obtaining intact fetal tissue is to dilate the woman's cervix to the point where the fetus could be extracted whole and alive. In some cases, reportedly, the fetus was dissected while still alive.[123]

Who is the primary patient in abortions involving fetal tissue procurement, the aborting woman or the possible recipient of the tissue? Salvaging intact fetal tissue requires that a fetus be delivered whole, but it is generally better for the woman if a fetus is fragmented in the womb. Will doctors determine the timing and methods of abortions to conform to the need for a certain kind of intact and/or usable fetal material?

Abortions should not become the handmaidens to other medical procedures such as fetal tissue transplants. This will increasingly happen, however, as abortions provide the fetal material for so-called miraculous medical research and treatment. In this case, women's right to abortion is increasingly made dependent on the need of others for fetal tissue, with women once more expected to be altruistic with what issues from their bodies.

Feminists and the Fetal Tissue Controversy

Most of the opposition to the use of fetal tissue has come from the conservative and religious right-wingers who strenuously oppose abortion.

Public debate over the use of fetal tissue has been stereotyped as a controversy between the forces of medical progress and the retrogressive right wing. No other side is represented in the debate, and the only recognized opponents are those who attack women's right to safe and legal abortion. Feminist objections are often lumped in with the right wing's, and, as in other areas, women and women's ideas are seen as derivative and having no independent status.

Conservatives and feminists base their arguments against the use of fetal tissue on very different grounds. The religious right is worried that abortions will increase due to medical research that requires increasingly more fetal tissue and that women will conceive for the express purpose of aborting fetuses to aid family members or for money. Feminists defend women's right to safe and legal abortion, but many fear that the current medical campaign for fetal tissue research and treatment will put pressure on certain groups of women to have abortions for family members or friends in need. It is also feared that other women, faced with making an abortion decision, might be persuaded directly or indirectly that "donating" fetal tissue redeems the abortion. With the increased opposition to abortion in the United States, even pro-choice advocates feel that abortions must be justified in some way, used for some benefit, and not "go to waste." A woman's decision to abort is increasingly made dependent on other considerations such as fetal tissue use. Abortion is a hard enough decision for many women to make, without being burdened with yet another decision of whether or not to donate fetal tissue.

Many feminists also contend that doctors who are eager to get good tissue samples must put women at additional risk of complications by altering the methods of abortion and by extending the time it takes to perform an abortion. Since there is disagreement over whether older or younger fetuses are more useful for fetal tissue transplants, feminists also point out that some women may be pressured into having later and riskier abortions in order to ensure intact fetuses with fully developed cells and tissues.

Ultimately, feminists ask, Where will all the embryos and fetal tissue come from? The number of elective abortions will never be enough for the amount of fetal tissue that doctors need, and it is a real possibility that the medical demand for fetal tissue could increase the trafficking in fetuses from Third World countries, rivaling the demand for babies, and be equally exploitative of women.

It is possible to believe in the morality of abortion and at the same time oppose the use of fetal tissue for commercial and medical purposes. Women have the right to safe, legal abortions, but women should not be fetal tissue providers. The fetus is not a person with rights, but the fetus is not simply a piece of tissue. Insisting on the moral, political, and legal rights of women to abortion does not mean that feminists and others have to surrender the fetal tissue controversy to the moral and political right.

Fetal tissue research and transplants cast women as mere environments and containers for the fetus. This has been the result of many reproductive technologies, in which women become "natural resources" whose bodies are mined for medical and scientific "gold." The role of women in this research is again she who provides the raw material. She is the resource for embryos, for eggs, for surrogate wombs, and now for fetal tissue—the field to be harvested or the cavern to be mined. Objections have been made by the political and religious right to harvesting the dead (fetuses) to help the living. Would that they had the same concern about harvesting living women.

More and more interventions into the prenatal area, such as performing surgery on fetuses or compelling a pregnant woman to undergo a cesarian after she has refused permission, are becoming common. Legal interventions to constrain women to have cesarians have been enforced by court order. One can imagine legal interventions to compel women undergoing abortion to give over fetuses for supposedly humanitarian research and treatment.

Objections to the commercializing of fetal tissue have been largely focused on blaming women, women who supposedly will be tempted to make money from conceiving and then aborting in order to sell the tissue. In this perspective, women are portrayed as the culprits who "conceive the idea of conceiving" for financial gain. Even a special advisory committee of the National Institutes of Health, which recommended that the federal government back medical research involving the use of fetal tissue, reserved one of its strongest warnings for women who, if paid, might be attracted to become pregnant just to conceive a fetus for abortion and research use.[124] Meanwhile, no one blames the medical world for generating and proliferating the supposed need for fetal tissue in all sorts of research.

The engine driving the need for fetal tissue is medical research— research into the diseases mentioned above but, increasingly, research for genetic engineering. Embryo experimentation is the area of medical research that is seldom mentioned when fetal research is discussed. More and more embryos/fetuses will be needed for more and more experimentation, particularly in the field of genetic engineering. In Europe, it is estimated that over 200,000 embryos are stockpiled in laboratories, prompting many doctors to be concerned about a world trade in accumulated embryos.[125] These numbers of stockpiled embryos are heading into the millions "because of the absence of controls over IVF clinics and scientists are reporting tales of secret experiments on excess embryos."[126]

This situation raises the question of the status of the fetus. Feminists have been reluctant to address the status of the fetus because, for one thing, the fetus has been raised to the level of person by the religious and political right, as women's personhood has come increasingly under attack. In fact, the legal trend has been to view *women in relation to the fetus* rather than the *fetus in relation to the pregnant woman*.[127] In controversies over abortion, fetal alcohol and drug syndromes, and doctor-ordered cesarians that conflict with the wishes of the pregnant woman, women are often viewed as reproductive criminals.

It is imperative that feminists especially begin to articulate the status of the fetus and situate the *fetus in relation to the pregnant woman*. A fetus is not a piece of tissue, nor is it analogous to another bodily organ like an eye or kidney. It is also not a person. Not an organ, not a person, it is unique and distinctively different from both. It *is*, however, an integral organism with developing human potential. Although a developing human being, it cannot develop outside the body of the pregnant woman. Since the fetus is unique and is uniquely situated in relation to the pregnant woman, the fetus cannot be given away as if it were an organ. The relation between a pregnant woman and her fetus is not a property or ownership relation. Putting it in more positive terms, and from the standpoint of the pregnant women, Catharine MacKinnon states that the fetus *is* both me and not me. It "is" the pregnant woman in the sense that it is in her and of her and is hers more than anyone's. It "is not" her in the sense that she is not all that is there.[128]

Thus the legal status of the fetus cannot be separated from the legal and social status of the pregnant woman in whose body it exists, and its existence is not that of personhood, certainly, but rather that of possibility.

Most women make decisions to abort faced with other crucial life concerns. Most women, in aborting, do not intend to devalue or use the fetus for any purpose. In contrast, fetal tissue is harvested from abortion clinics expressly for its utilitarian value—for research and for medical treatment of others. The "intentionality" of this harvesting, that is, the reasons for which fetal salvaging is done, is quite different from the abortion procedure itself, which does not require the abortion *and* the fetus to be utilized for another purpose.

Because fetal remains are fragmented, they are typically portrayed as medical waste to be salvaged for intact tissue and used in the noble pursuit of curing incurable diseases. However, fetal remains are not waste; they are simply "remains" and should simply "remain." They should not be part of routine salvaging expeditions such as fetal tissue processing. This is not to say that they should be accorded a ceremony such as a burial, but that they remain unused. Rummaging through the fetal remains and portraying those remains as waste border on a scavenging operation in which fetuses are devalued and objectified for their use value in the same way that other parts and products of women's bodies, such as uteri and eggs, are externalized, used, and commodified.

Regulation: The Illusory Answer

Currently the human tissue industry is largely unregulated. Even its size and extent are unknown. Many people think that the whole matter of fetal tissue can be regulated to take care of the concerns raised in this chapter. Regulations have been proposed: to ensure that women give informed consent to the procedure; to ban the sale of fetal tissue; to ensure that fetal dissection cannot take place while fetuses are still alive; to separate doctors performing abortions from those using the fetal tissue; to prevent women from designating beneficiaries of fetal tissue; and to confine research and treatment with fetal tissue to quality controlled medical centers.

A system of regulation that would allow fetuses to be used for medical research and treatment begins a process that is likely to end with the widespread use of fetal remains for a variety of purposes—experimental, therapeutic, and commercial. The line between therapeutic and commercial blurs when, for example, human fetal remains are transferred from clinics to tissue processors to medical labs and transplant centers—for a price, a processing fee, a rental fee for clinic space, or a "reimbursement" for each tissue sample. The line blurs even further if, as one critical journal speculated, human fetal remains were found to be a safe, nonpolluting, highly effective and efficient fertilizer capable of exponentially increasing world crop harvests. Medical treatment today, world hunger treatment tomorrow. Why *not* other humanitarian uses of fetal remains?[129]

As with surrogacy, powerful interests are likely to become vested in how this industry is organized and regulated. The pattern that has emerged in attempts to regulate other reproductive technologies and arrangements such as surrogacy is that those who have the most to gain from such regulation are those who are at the forefront of influencing and crafting the direction of legislation.

The incentive for legal regulation of fetal tissue is coming from the medical profession and the fetal tissue processors, not from the women directly involved. This is a far different context from the one in which the impetus for abortion legislation emerged. Abortion was fought for by women. Fetal tissue regulation is being driven by the processing agencies and the medical research community.

A *Wall Street Journal* reporter suggested that "a transplant industry based upon fetal-tissue technology could dwarf the present organ-transplant industry."[130] In addition, *The Progressive* commented,

> The pharmaceutical and medical-supply corporations will enter the picture. . . . One company, now in the development stages, plans to begin marketing cells grown from fetal tissue within a few years. While it says it uses tissue strictly from "third-party, non-profit procuring agencies," that could change as more and more tissue is needed to supply the expected demand.[131]

The only chilling effect on the use of fetal tissue for medical research was the decision of the former Bush administration to impose a ban on federally funded fetal tissue transplants into humans. Former secretary of Health and Human Services, Louis Sullivan, rejected the conclusions of a 1988 NIH advisory committee that recommended continuing clinical trials with fetal tissue. Instead, the Bush administration decided that "permitting the human fetal research at issue will increase the incidence of abortion across the country."[132] It was primarily this decision that linked the fetal tissue debate with the controversy over abortion, collapsing the two. And ever since then, most liberals appear to be defending fetal tissue research and transplants, almost as a knee-jerk response to this linkage.

In April 1991 the U.S. House of Representatives Subcommittee on Health and the Environment held public hearings on H.R. 1532, a bill to reauthorize the National Institutes of Health. As part of the congressional reauthorization of NIH, this bill called for overturning the Bush ban on fetal tissue research and transplantation. It also was intended to bar the executive branch from imposing any such prohibition on the Department of Health and Human Services in the future, and it would have released federal monies for fetal tissue research.

I appeared before the House subcommittee as the only witness to testify, for many of the reasons cited in this chapter, against this bill.[133] Various representatives from Parkinson's patients' groups, a woman with Parkinson's disease, and two parents of children with a rare genetic disease called Hurler's syndrome all testified in favor of the bill. In a medical first, the two parents, along with their transplant surgeon, reported the results of a new fetus-to-fetus tissue surgery that was performed in the womb. They declared that their infant, who was born in November 1990 appears to be in good health, but that it is still too early to tell if he will survive. Interestingly, these parents testified that they were adamantly opposed to abortion yet had decided that it was ethical to use tissue from an aborted fetus.

All of the witnesses in favor of lifting the ban testified on the presumption that the research was progressive, proven to be therapeutic, and life saving. None questioned its claims or seemed aware of the skepticism and caution advocated by many in the scientific community. None of those in favor of lifting the ban, including all the liberal congressmen on the subcommittee, addressed the consequences *to women* of fetal tissue research and transplantation. All of the Democrats supporting the research appeared to acquiesce in the sentiment that abortions were a waste if the fetal tissue obtained from them were not put to medical use. And one of the first acts of President Clinton during the initial week of assuming the presidency was to lift the Bush ban on fetal tissue research and transplantation, giving the go-ahead to fetal tissue utilization.

When testifying before the House subcommittee on Health and Environment, I stated that although the bill under consideration, H.R. 1532, limited the more flagrant abuses that are present and possible with the use of fetal tissue, it would open up a hornet's nest by giving the legal go-ahead to a *system* of routinely harvesting fetal tissue. Although the proposed legislation closes some of the glaring loopholes now present in the unregulated world of fetal tissue procurement, it also gives that world a stable marketing and research environment. Thus by regulating fetal tissue procurement and transplants, their availability will be increased. In addition, the very availability of a technology ensures its use. As with other new technologies, many physicians will feel compelled to provide fetal tissue to their patients. As the report on "Human Rights Aspects of Transactions in Body Parts and Human Fetuses" that was prepared for UNESCO recognized, doctors are indeed advocates of technologies in which they specialize, and thus these technologies such as fetal tissue transplants reflect that demonstrable interest. "As part of a technological 'subculture of objectivity' many [physicians] feel a moral imperative to use all available new technologies with their patients while others admit the lure of using them to bring new excitement to their practices."[134]

Conclusion

All technology is not automatically progress. Regulating a technology does not ensure that a technology will be used in a progressive way. Regulation does not address the international trafficking potential for fetal tissue or the casting of women in the role of human incubators. There can be no exploitation of fetuses or children without a prior exploitation of women, from whence fetuses and children come.

The situation of women and children is very much connected; this is a biological but, more significantly, a political fact. Both women and children share in the same kinds of sexual abuse, and increasingly both become commodities on the international reproductive market. Both are subject increasingly to medical experimentation. New reproductive arrangements, such as surrogacy, are increasing the traffic in women and children across national borders. Women are the breeders; children are the product bred. We have here the international harvesting of women and children.

Many U.S. Americans recognize the horrors of the child organ and illegal adoption trade. Yet they approve of legislation legalizing and/or regulating surrogate contracts, without seeing any connection between the former and the latter. Surrogacy is the acceptable face of reproductive trafficking, yet there is little distinction between a domestic and an intercountry market in women and children. What we call surrogacy in the West is a variant on baby selling abroad. One is soft-core exploitation, the other hard-core. One is glossy, the other graphic. The only distinction is that in surrogacy, the father buys his own genetic child and thereby confers legitimacy on surrogate arrangements because the child is recognized as "his."

The reproductive trafficking in women and children contains all the worst elements of human rights violations. It involves the purchase and sale of human beings, coercion, the uprooting of women and children frequently from their countries of origin and from their culture, sometimes the torture of both, often the medical violation of both, and, more often than we know, the death of both. The reproductive exploitation of women and children, along with their sexual exploitation, is an act of total denigration of human beings. Until we recognize such sexual, reproductive, and medical practices as violations of human rights and abolish the overall structure of this international trafficking in women and children, nothing will change.

CHAPTER SIX

International Human Rights, Integrity, and Legal Frameworks

The articulation of reproductive rights has been mired in proprietary language. The right to control one's body too often frames the body as a possession and as capital to dispose of as the individual wishes. This view of rights analogizes the body to private property. To say I *own* my body is substantively different from saying I *am* my body. In the latter articulation, the body becomes more than a private space that the person is free to do with as she pleases. It becomes the ground of the self that has integrity, dignity, and worth—more than a use value.

Theories about owning the body help objectify and commodify women's bodies, both for others and the woman herself, creating a distance between a woman's self and a woman's body. A *proprietary right* to my body allows me to submit it to the control of others or to do with it what I please, no matter how those actions undermine not only my dignity, my integrity, and my ability to act but also the dignity, integrity, and abilities of others as well. A *substantive right* to my body means the body is more than a mere possession and raises the fundamental issue of the relationship between my body and my self, and my self to the class of women worldwide.

Prostitution and surrogacy are based on the notion that a man can buy or rent a woman's body, as in a market exchange or real estate transaction, and that a woman has the right to sell or rent her own body for money. The body, however, is not property, and therefore it is not transferable in a market sense. Yet reproductive liberalism, in North America, is locked into an oppressive legal language and reality of rights that derives from a male-dominant tradition of property rights, which institutionalizes a female body as a possession.

As we have seen throughout this book, property rights stem from a liberal individualist tradition that does very little to protect the rights of some individuals against other individuals, for example, the rights of so-called surrogates when they come into conflict with the rights of ejaculatory fathers. German feminist Maria Mies has made the significant point that even the individual, in the liberal individualist tradition of rights, is vivisected. "If the *individual*—the undivided person—has been divided up into her/his saleable parts, the individual has disappeared. There is only the *dividual* which can be further divided up."[1] Following this logic, she asks how autonomy or rights can apply to an individual who is a dividual and thus has no designated subject. Even a subject is necessary for the buying and selling of body parts.

> But this subject, this person, has been eliminated in theory *and* in practice. What is left is an assembly of parts. *The bourgeois individual has eliminated itself.* Hence, we understand why there is no longer a place for ethical questions, neither within the individual body nor within the societal body.[2]

Within the long history of rights discourse, rights have also been essentialized as "natural" rights. Natural rights have historically been used in both conservative and radical defenses of what is perceived as given in the human condition. The right to procreate has been conceived as a natural right, and, by extension, technological reproduction has been recently promoted as the means to fulfill one's natural right to procreate. Thus the male-dominant tradition of property rights converges with a version of natural rights proclaiming a natural right to procreate, a natural right to a child, a natural right to use any means necessary to procreate, and thereby a natural right to use any person necessary to procreate.

When procreation is defined as a natural right, it is viewed as deriving from a natural instinct, comparable to eating and sleeping. Attempts

to institutionalize procreation as a natural right divest the person pro-
creating of moral responsibility, so that anything a man or woman does
to reproduce is treated as an instinctive response beyond the control of
human will and human relations. One way that the right to procreate
becomes a law of nature is that, as a right, it becomes grounded in a natural need, that is, a compelling paternal urge or maternal instinct that
demands an outlet. The right to procreate, portrayed as a natural right,
renaturalizes motherhood and reproduction and grounds men's rights
to "their" children in the natural order.

The challenge is to recognize the material contribution that women
make to reproduction and pregnancy while at the same time not essentializing that contribution as natural female destiny. The challenge is
also to argue that this contribution alone does not constitute the primary action or agency of female reproduction but grounds, in unique
ways, the relationship of woman to fetus. The challenge is not to expand
men's already prevalent rights over women's bodies by reinstitutional-
izing male "genetic fulfillment" as a justification for reproductive technologies and contracts.

It has long been the task of feminism to challenge the natural and
show it to be political. Reproductive behavior, like any other behavior,
can and must be subject to an analysis embedded in human social and
political relations.

Feminist Challenges to Rights Theory

The theories of choice, privacy, and procreative liberty promote rights
that are substantively bankrupt and in which anything can be asserted
as a right. Within che framework of individual rights, every desire and
preference is phr..ied as a right; in the world of new reproductive technologies and contracts, the language of rights is used to promote and
sell reproductive products and persons. Therefore, some feminists are
advocating that we stop talking about rights and instead talk about power
or justice or, in Maria Mies's term, "the re-creation of living relations."

In a discussion of pornography, activists Deborah Cameron and
Liz Fraser contend that it is women's power, not rights, that should be
the issue. "Feminists must struggle for power. . . . If we don't have this

clear—and we demand 'rights'—we are forced into arenas where we cannot, by definition, win the battle."[3] To continue using the language of rights, they maintain, associates women with a liberalism that has proven to be ineffective in protecting women's lives.

Human rights educator Sherene Razack also challenges rights thinking. In an article entitled "Wrong Rights: Feminism Applied to Law," she explains that much of the work she did as a human rights educator addressed the daily realities of oppression in the language of rights. Although formerly she insisted that the rights of women be honored by providing women with the means to these rights, she now disputes that framework. "It is from rights-thinking that we get that curious abstraction of the fetus without a womb. Sooner or later, we have to expose rights-based perspectives, dressed as they usually are in abstractions, for what they are: a poorly disguised way of preserving things just as they are."[4]

Maria Mies eloquently criticizes the reproductive rights focus of the "Reproductive Laws for the 1990s" project in which Lori Andrews, especially, lays out a superficial market-based theory and property version of reproductive rights for women.[5] Mies also criticizes the reproductive rights framework of the "Global Network on Reproductive Rights," which not only "transform[s] questions of reproduction and sexuality into legal problems, but maintain[s] the idea of individual self-determination of each woman as the essence of our emancipatory hopes."[6]

In the United States, the Critical Legal Studies (CLS) school has advanced one of the most well-known arguments against rights discourse and theory. Their position is premised on the assumption that talk of rights is harmful because rights are often pitted against larger issues of social need. Therefore, they maintain, instead of arguing on behalf of *rights* of the homeless, for example, we should be talking about the *needs* of the homeless. Further, CLS argues that rights "have only the meaning that power wishes them to have."[7]

In responding particularly to the position of CLS, African American legal scholar Patricia Williams counters, "For the historically disempowered, the conferring of rights is symbolic of all the denied aspects of their humanity: rights imply a respect that places one in the referential range of self and others, that elevates one's status *from human*

body to social being."[8] "From human body to social being" is particularly relevant also to women's quest for sexual and reproductive justice.
For it is here too that "the attainment of rights signifies the respectful
behavior, the collective responsibility, properly owed by a society to one
of its own." Putting rights discourse in a larger ethical framework, Williams reminds us that, for Blacks, the prospect of attaining full rights has
been "fiercely motivational," a "source of hope," and rooted in "the sanc-
tity of one's own personal boundaries."[9]

Against the critics of rights discourse, Williams argues that it is not
the assertion of rights but the failure of rights commitment that has
led to, for example, the history of African American slavery in the
United States. Therefore, when critical legal theorists argue that we
should abandon rights discourse and theory, they are arguing from the
vantage point of those who already have such rights and whose rights
have not been abridged. African Americans know only too well that the
Bill of Rights was shaped by white slaveholders to protect their im-
peratives and that the sparse enforcement of civil rights provisions is
but a mere sop, given the history of Black enslavement on all levels.
But, at the same time, it is Blacks who nonetheless continue to insist
on those rights, fueled by years of existing in "a world without any
meaningful boundaries . . . the crushing weight of total—bodily and
spiritual—*intrusion.*"[10]

In contrast to the critics of rights discourse and theory, I would
echo "the crushing weight of total—bodily and spiritual—intrusion" that
has burdened women under a system of reproductive technologies and
contracts. As I see it, the task is not to discard rights but to ground them
in power, justice, self-determination, and international relations. These
international human rights are grounded in the dignity of the individual
and the integrity of relations between individuals and groups in society.
Because so much of women's sexual and reproductive inequality centers
on violations of bodily integrity, physical self-determination, and personal and social dignity, taking for granted that women are inferior in
human worth, these principles are hardly symbolic considerations.

My work is grounded not only in a woman's individual bodily integrity but in the *integrity of the living relations among women.* Both
aspects of women's integrity have been assaulted by postmodernist
theory and practice. Postmodernism decenters the individual subject

and decenters relations among different women, using difference to devitalize rather than to enliven. Postmodernist theory and practice have also decentered the ethical in the sense of regarding principles such as the dignity or integrity of a woman's person as without any determinate meaning. Since there is no stabilizing center such as truth, conscience, or integrity of being, the ethical dimension vaporizes. Everything is text and more text, signs and more signs, signifiers and more signifiers, encouraging endless rounds of self-devouring equivocations.

The postmodernist decentering of the ethical is comparable to a liberal conception of rights that increasingly dismisses principles such as a woman's bodily integrity or dignity as symbolic. Choice, procreative liberty, and privacy are based on a supposed hard, objective, and quantitative analytical core of legal reasoning, while principles such as the integrity of a woman's body and the dignity of a woman's life are downgraded to "soft" value judgments on the periphery of law. Legal scholar John Robertson, for example, reduces such principles to "moral judgments," "an affront to moral sensibilities," and an "aesthetic revulsion" that cannot be allowed to interfere with people's freedom to procreate.[11] Feminist ethics is relegated to the soft sand of the ethical playground, not comparable to the "hard-on" standards of legal positivism and quantifiable public policy.

The right to privacy is an especially good example of how the U.S. controversy over technological reproduction is shaped by a language of rights that is more legislative and policy oriented than politically and ethically substantive. This appeal to privacy puts the issue of reproductive rights beyond considerations of social justice and social ethics. Moral claims, which assert that a surrogate contract, for example, violates the dignity or bodily integrity of women, as well as social justice claims that women who are economically disadvantaged are exploited in surrogacy and that surrogacy helps create a breeder class of women, are considered beside the point. Individual liberty becomes more important than justice for all, and individual claims more palpable than moral and social claims.

At the same time that I criticize liberal individual rights positivism, however, I am unwilling to give over a theory of individualism to the liberals, thereby dismissing any individualism as counterproductive. The work of many women often appears as "merely individualistic" because of the ways in which women have had to assert themselves on an individual level. In this view, women's individual acts of resistance are not seen as challenging the capitalist state. Within a bourgeois liberal culture, however, women's claims to individuality have been strangled by a biological or ontological essentialism that consigns women to the realm of nature. Paradoxically, the first task of any essentialized *group* is to assert the *individuality* of its members.

Because historically women have been submerged in the generic totalitarianism of an essentialism that has perceived and treated us as nonindividuals, it is imperative to establish the value of female self-determination as a basis for right relations. In fact, I would argue that Maria Mies's idea of the "re-creation of living relations," what I call right relations, must be grounded in female self-determination. However, this claim to female self-determination, and other individual claims or rights, must not be asserted outside of, or in opposition to, the living relations among women. When surrogacy is valorized as an individual woman's right to control her own body, it ignores these relations among women, that is, it ignores what happens when one woman's claim to control her own body results in women as a group—especially economically and racially disadvantaged women—being treated as breeders for others. When a woman's right to do whatever she wants to do with her body is valorized as feminism, feminism is stripped of its collective content and becomes little more than an individual woman's ability to adapt herself to the bourgeois image of the self-centered man.

The U.S. tradition of rights is grounded in the atomized individual and lacks any ethical grounding in the integrity or dignity of the individual and the group. In contrast, every international declaration of human rights is based on the dignity and integrity of the individual in society. Therefore, whatever violates a person's dignity or integrity—economic exploitation, medical experimentation, and the trafficking in women's bodies for sexual or reproductive purposes—is not a right, either for the person who says they choose to engage in these acts or for those who induce them to participate.

It is my goal in this final chapter to develop a theory of human rights and technological justice for women, grounded in the dignity and integrity of a woman's person but set in the context of international rights relations.

International Human Rights

There have been many attempts to develop standards for judging medical violations of human rights, the major ones being the Nuremberg Code and the Helsinki Declaration (revised several times). Other human rights documents and conventions that apply to the area of medical practice are: the International Covenant on Civil and Political Rights; the 1948 Convention condemning genocide; the 1949 Convention on suppressing trafficking in prostitutes and similar forms of slavery; the 1952 Convention on the political rights of women, as well as the later Declaration and Convention on the Elimination of All Forms of Discrimination against Women (1967; 1981); the 1965 Convention on the Elimination of All Forms of Racial Discrimination; the 1984 Convention outlawing torture; and the 1985 Declaration on the Use of Scientific and Technological Progress in the Interests of Peace and for the Benefit of Mankind. It is not my intention to recount all the specific principles in these documents that can be applied to an analysis of technological justice for women but rather to emphasize certain broader principles of these human rights documents.

In contrast to the Bill of Rights and the U.S. Constitution, all international human rights documents are rooted in the concept of human dignity.[12] The claim to human dignity has been made in every formal articulation of international human rights. Although opinions differ as to what dignity entails, the basic idea is articulated in the preamble to the Universal Declaration of Human Rights, which begins with the principle that the equal and inalienable rights of everyone are grounded in "the inherent dignity of . . . all members of the human family." This dignity must be recognized as "the foundation of freedom, justice and peace in the world." Article 1 of the declaration reaffirms, "All human beings are born free and equal in dignity and rights."

Conceptions of dignity differ, especially between the West and the East. Many have criticized the individualism of the Human Rights Declaration, contending that it grounds human rights in a Western theory of rights in such a way that greed becomes self-sacrifice and selfishness becomes altruism. As ethicist Warren Lee Holleman has written,

> We grant individuals a plethora of rights and freedoms. We glamorize the lone pioneers who challenge the frontiers of medicine, outer

space, and the Wild West. We idolize the rare rugged individualists and Horatio Algers who succeed when the odds are against them. We put "blind faith" in the "invisible hand" of the free enterprise system, believing that as individuals pursue their own profit-maximizing activities the "invisible hand" of the market will work all things together for the good of all persons. We believe that egotistic impulses somehow serve the common good, thus we justify them.[13]

This is also an apt description of the way that new reproductive technologies and surrogacy have been justified as rights by the reproductive liberals. Reproductive liberals accent atomistic individualism and distrust political institutions, most specifically the state, which they view as interfering with the procreative liberty of individuals in restricting new reproductive technologies.

In contrast, many developing countries have pointed out that it is not always the rights of *all* individuals that are in need of protection from the state. For example, many people in Third World countries are faced with tremendous poverty and hunger. This is not caused by governments restricting the freedom of individuals per se but rather by governments allowing a certain class of individuals to flourish at the expense of others. Thus it is important to consider which classes or groups of individuals are in need of rights. This can only be done if the material differences, that is, the specific inequalities of certain individuals in relation to others, are incorporated into visions and declarations of human rights. For women, this means talking about gender inequality.

Failure to make tangible the ideals of freedom and dignity for specific women in society means these ideals will be expressed in abstract, Western, and male terms. What then prevails is a liberal democratic individualism in which anarchistic individual tastes, preferences, and options become known as rights and in which the supposedly heroic actions of the masculinist individual setting himself in opposition to the masculinist state becomes the human rights drama, for example, the scientist as hero who develops reproductive technologies in opposition to state regulation of research and treatment. The fact that male individuals and interests also assert themselves against female individuals and interests is swallowed up by the portrayal of the civil libertarian male as a hero resisting state repression of so-called individual liberties.

Human rights violations get ignored in the new reproductive technological context, because what male individuals do to female individuals is *not defined as a violation, but rather as a civil liberty* (for example, to enter into a surrogate contract or to submit one's body to exploitative medical treatment). Any state intervention to protect women from exploitation is seen as a restriction on individual liberties, privacy, and rights, not as a legal safeguard for women from reproductive violation. The male entitlement to a woman's body is rationalized as a woman's reproductive right. The male right to genetic fulfillment and continuity is reworked as a woman's right to sign a surrogate contract or subject herself to an experimental IVF procedure, rather than her right not to be placed in the situation of surrogacy and her right not to be subjected to experimental procedures, even when some women supposedly choose to do so.

Liberalism has perverted individualism and used it to promote a masculinist consumerist philosophy and practice. Liberalism replaces a politics of resistance to male domination with the so-called freedom of enlightened self-interest for men and for some women. Liberal individualism reifies the male individual, ascribing to him fundamental, absolute, and unlimited rights. It grounds everything in the unchecked right of the male individual to absolute liberty of property, pleasure, and now reproductive fulfillment. And what it gives to men, it pretends to give to women.

Critics of the human rights movement have asserted that Western human rights advocates do not hold basic human needs and material entitlements as rights equal to civil liberties ("food versus freedom"). As one critic wrote, "To have freedom of speech and assembly while living in squalor is as inimical to human dignity as is living in relative economic security while being denied fundamental rights of self-expression."[14]

The same deficiency exists in the current liberal version of reproductive rights. Based on the civil libertarian model of rights, women have the so-called civil liberty of entering into a surrogate contract, while their basic human need of dignified and economically sustaining work is denied. It is the right to dignified and economically sustaining work, not the right to become a surrogate, that contributes to women's genuine empowerment. Surrogacy, promoted as a woman's reproductive right, keeps a woman in the state of personal devaluation, systematic subordination, relegating her to the work of breeding and to being defined as a reproductive instrument. It is absurd to assume that a woman should be provided with the right to enter prostitution, pornography, or surrogacy, without providing her with the means to go beyond these so-called rights.

On Being Gender Specific

Human rights groups, such as Amnesty International, have not until recently focused on the abuses done to women as women and on the gender-specific risks faced by women in situations of political imprisonment and torture.[15] Outside the narrowly defined categories of political torture and imprisonment, however, other modes of torture, such as medical violation and nonstate imprisonment, for example, the domestic incarceration and abuse of women or sexual slavery and reproductive servitude, have not received independent recognition by human rights groups. These women have not been the subject of human rights investigations unless they have somehow come under the rubric of state-defined political human rights violations. This ignores the fact that women are the major battleground of human rights abuse, as promoted by the state and by nonstate male supremacy, such as medical research interests.[16] It must be recognized that violations of women's human rights often take place outside the context of state torture and political repression. Gender-specific human rights recognizes the wider context of female subordination in which women live.

Any declaration of rights must be supplemented by a declaration of relations—relations of individuals to each other, which include obligations, responsibilities, and connections. Rights are not meaningful unless they specify the relations between individuals—between men and women, and between women and women. Human rights must be stated in gender-specific and enforceable terms, else they die the death of vague ideals.

The development of new reproductive technologies and contracts cannot be divorced from the systems that enforce women's sexual and reproductive inequality in our global society. Reproductive technologies must be seen in their totality, not just as helping someone to have a child, but within the larger context of women's political inequality and the systematic subordination that has disadvantaged women in every sphere. This includes economic poverty and discrimination, demeaning work and prostitution, political disenfranchisement, sexual abuse, battery, rape, forced reproduction, lack of access to education, devaluation of talent and ability, and exclusion from the public sphere.

Any valorizing of reproductive technologies as help for the infertile only helps sentimentalize women's inequality. It dismisses, at the outset, gender-specific questions, such as: Why do women bear the burden of these painful, unhealthy, and risky techniques? Why are women in the West channeled into motherhood at any cost to themselves? Why are women in the Third World channeled out of motherhood at any cost to themselves? Why do these procedures demand that women adapt to ever more demeaning and exploitative treatment? Why do these technologies reify the image of Western women as reproductive environments for the fetus? Why do these technologies reify the image of Third World women as population polluters?

Gender-specific ethics means that moral meaning and public policy should be guided by the presence of gender specificity. To be more concrete, it means that any assessment of reproductive technologies takes as its ethical starting point the question of women's status and how the technology enhances or diminishes gender inequality. Gender-specific ethics devotes primary attention to, in this case, a technology's consequences for women. It recognizes not only the harm, but the devaluation that happens to all women when some women are used as breeders, reproductive commodities, population polluters, and test sites for new drugs and technologies. Thus it sets these technologies in the context of relations among women, recognizing that women who do not necessarily use the technologies are affected by them.

In *Feminism Unmodified: Discourses on Life and Law*, Catharine MacKinnon develops this notion of gender specificity as a foundation for legislation. Gender specificity recognizes "the most sex-differential abuses of women as a gender" and the reality that these abuses are not mere sex "differences" but "a socially situated subjection of women."[17]

Gender specificity also means that treating women and men as the same in law, as if all things are equal at the starting point, is merely gender neutrality. Most bioethical analyses of reproductive technologies proceed as if these techniques are gender neutral. These analyses thus obfuscate the gendered relations of social power that are manifested in all aspects of reproductive technologies. A gender-specific ethics and public policy will confront the degradation of women in the so-called private sphere of reproduction and will recognize the gender inequality that exists as a result, for example, of prescriptive motherhood and societal sanctions for infertile women.

MacKinnon's work on gender specificity, especially the way she has developed difference versus dominance in law, is both ground breaking and insightful. Where I would add to, and perhaps diverge from, her theory is in emphasizing the *ethical underpinnings* of law and public policy. Where MacKinnon has stated that pornography, for example, is "not a moral issue,"[18] I would argue that pornography is indeed a moral issue—not an issue of morality as circumscribed by the right-wing fundamentalists, that is, reducible to moralisms about obscenity, but rather an issue of what Andrea Dworkin has called moral intelligence and Alice Walker, the "rigors of discernment." MacKinnon contends that "the feminist critique of pornography is a politics, specifically politics from women's point of view, meaning the standpoint of the subordination of women to men. Morality here means good and evil; pornography is a political practice."[19] While I agree with this notion of the political, it is a partial definition. Political issues are ethical too, and unless we seek to rejoin the ethical and the political, values such as the dignity or integrity of a woman's body have no *political meaning* and politics has no ethical grounding.

Rejoining the Ethical and the Political

The history of sexual and reproductive liberalism has helped reinforce the tendency, present in the history of modern philosophy and social theory, to sever ethics from politics and, most recently, from law. If ethics and politics are to be rejoined and form the grounding for law and public policy, reproductive self-determination must be viewed as a substantive *moral*, public policy, and legislative issue. This means that appeals to the dignity of a woman's person and a woman's claim to bodily integrity become the centerpiece rather than the periphery of legal reasoning.

This also means that we must reassess the meaning of the ethical and its severance from social justice, politics, and law. Progressive and feminist circles show a certain distrust of, even hostility toward, ethical analysis. This distrust and hostility have resulted, in part, from the identification of morality with male-dominant morality and with the moral fundamentalism of the religious right. This simplistic equation of morality with moralism and with moral fundamentalism has to be challenged, lest we too quickly and uncritically concede the ethical realm to the moral fundamentalists.

In addition, postmodernism treats conscience as a pretextual, vestigial organ, labeling it as an outmoded centering of subjectivity. In this view, we are encouraged to overcome the vestiges of any moral intelligence left over from the Pleistocene ethical age in which moral responsibility is viewed as a rock in the head—something like a crystallized residue remaining from an earlier epoch. In contrast to postmodernism's decentering of the ethical, I argue for ethical analysis as an act of expressed and committed political judgment, not mere rhetorical practice.

An adequate feminist politics needs the depth and value of a moral passion and purpose. A strong politics of feminism should not force women out of the ethical domain because that domain has been colonized and defined by men. Moral intelligence and moral passion are the most vital resources that an oppressed group has. Such intelligence and passion form the groundswell of power, since without them the political loses its moorings all too easily.

The emphasis on a one-dimensional view of politics in political theory and practice has de-ethicized issues of power. When power is de-ethicized, decisions often get made from, for example, a cost-benefit or purely consequentialist calculus. And when politics is disjoined from ethics, politics frequently gets reduced to policy. Values are reduced to symbolic considerations.

Citing philosopher Alisdair MacIntyre's observation that the original sense of the term *value* was monetary, philosopher Caroline Whitbeck points out that only later did value acquire its more ethical sense.

One result of this original definition of value is that metaphors drawn from economics have dominated our thinking and judgment about "issues of value (the good). . . . Within the framework of classical Liberal theory it is assumed that values can be *ordered* and even *quantified* and *maximized.*"[20] Liberal methods for evaluating and judging, from the utilitarian calculus to the present-day use of decision analysis, are often taken from economics. Thus the major ethical task has been to order and balance competing claims, not to make value discernments.

In a similar manner, environmental engineer H. Patricia Hynes talks about the reduction of environmental goals to green consumerism. Environmental objectives, such as clean air or clean water, and other matters of environmental justice are costed out in market values or get analyzed primarily in a cost-benefit framework. Hynes takes note of a trend in the area of resource economics "to reduce natural systems, the functions of nature, and even the right to pollute, to market commodities whose value is based on human consumption or willingness-to-pay. In this brand of neo-classical economics, the value of a mountain is calculated by polling people on how much they would pay to hike it."[21]

Similarly, reproductive liberalism has spawned a neoclassical idea that reduces procreative choice to reproductive consumerism, where women and children are the reproductive commodities and men the reproductive consumers. Reproductive consumerism nowhere addresses the commodification of women and children or the connections between Western reproductive technological development and Third World trafficking in women, children, fetuses, and body parts. Much less does it address the male-dominant values that generate reproductive consumerism—for example, men's so-called need for genetic progeny. And even less does it address issues of the violation of the integrity of a woman's body and how this violation affects other women who are then seen and treated as breeders or population polluters.

Science and technology must be used to enhance human dignity, not to demean it, as has happened with the new technologies of reproduction, which are invasive, fragmenting, and often destructive to women's health and well-being. Ethical claims shift the ground beneath law and public policy. They determine what gives them life and, ultimately, what imbues law and public policy. Feminist politics must be grounded in this kind of ethical and moral intelligence, else we end up with a superficial and decentered concept and practice of rights.

Recentering the Subject: On the Need for an Ethic of the Dignity and Integrity of Women

Feminist ethics can restore a *teleology* to feminist politics. Where politics and political activity can be distorted by the emphasis on the means, ethics revives the emphasis on *ends*—in the context of technological reproduction, *the value of women as ends in themselves, independent of reproductive worth.* As reproductive technologies and contracts proliferate, women are increasingly viewed as means to another's fulfillment, health, well-being, or population goals. In fetal tissue research, abortions become the handmaidens to the salvaging of fetal tissue for medical use; in surrogacy women are hired wombs contracted for procreative use; in IVF, wives are used to bear children, often for husbands who have infertility problems and thus cannot procreate naturally and normally or because of the societal prescription that women must reproduce at any cost to themselves.

The new reproductive technologies reinforce the perception that, apart from their ability to procreate, women have no independent or intrinsic value. An ethics of integrity asserts that women are *ends* in themselves with dignity and integrity of person, that is, women are independent, integral beings, not breeders. This seems to be a quaint notion in an age where it increasingly becomes difficult for women to define the limits of what must be endured and sacrificed in many situations: for a pregnancy; for not becoming pregnant; for fetal benefit; for medical research and the conquest of disease; and for unrelated men who must have "their own" biological children. The new reproductive technologies reinforce the conditional value of women in medical treatment, law, and public policy. Woman's independent integrity is set aside.

Integrity is not intangible; it has a material reality. It is socioeconomic as well as existential, physical as well as spiritual. It includes a woman's work and health as well as her needs and beliefs, all of which should not be subordinated to reproduction. In the whole debate over reproductive technologies, few talk about women's own need for bodily

and spiritual integrity. Technological reproduction and surrogacy promote the view that medical research, male genetic fulfillment, women's
supposed desperate need to have children, as well as the creeping perception and validation of the fetus as independent person or patient
have more integrity than a woman has in her own person. Women, in
contrast, have no value, independent of and unconditioned by sexuality
and reproduction. Western women have come to be seen as *owing* children to themselves, to their male partners, and to those with whom they
have signed a contract. And women in developing countries have come
to be seen as either *owing* children they cannot care for to the Western
world, who can, or as targets/acceptors of population control and contraceptive drug testing. In the reproductive realm, others' interests
have become paramount, and what a woman owes to herself, independent of her ability to procreate, is ignored.

This lack of integrity has graphic consequences for women's health
and well-being. When multiple tests, technological interventions, and
drug cocktails are an *intrinsic* part of new reproductive treatment,
these treatments undermine, in a most physical way, women's self-
determination. A woman's life, work, and health are demoted when they
do not mesh with her reproductive worth. Next to procreation, reinforced in Western technological reproduction as women's greatest
need, these other needs are perceived as trivial.

The new reproductive technologies reflect a view of women as
decentered subjects and social beings. The material outcome of such
a view is a concrete carving up of women into body parts, specifically,
into wombs, eggs, and follicles. But the worst thing about this decentering of woman as subject is that a woman is divided from her own perceptions of herself, of her own body and of her issue. As one so-called
surrogate phrased it, "I'm only baby-sitting for their child." In addition,
surrogacy decenters motherhood into categories of genetic, gestational,
and social. What better way of dividing women from themselves and
each other?

Recentering women as subjects—individual subjects with bodily
integrity, and subjects with other women in resistance to male dominance *and* in relation to each other—is the radical feminist challenge
to the postmodernist decentering of the female body and spirit, and
to the disintegration of women's dignity and integrity inherent in new

reproductive procedures. Integrity and dignity are at once transcendent and concrete values. Unless integrity is recognized in terms of women's particular needs, actions, and relationships, it is little more than an empty notion—"nonsense upon stilts," as the eighteenth-century philosopher Bentham phrased it.

In an age of technological reproduction and commodified reproductive contracts, women need a principle that goes beyond reproductive freedom. Any concept of rights, as a cluster of claims made by women for social justice, must derive its principal moral warrant from the concept of integrity. The right to bodily integrity is particularly grounded in women's history since it is women in all countries who have been abused sexually and reproductively through the body. For women, the principle of bodily integrity is not intangible or symbolic but very historical, material, and cross-cultural. The ultimate tragedy of technological reproduction is that women are made to negate their own bodies, treating their bodies as instruments for their own or someone else's reproductive goals and splitting their bodies from their selves.

Regulation Versus Abolition

As a legal approach to technological and contractual reproduction, many have advocated regulation, that is, encumbering new reproductive technologies and arrangements with certain legal restrictions and bringing them more within the purview of state and/or federal guidelines. Many reproductive rights groups have cited the dangers of these technologies for women but nonetheless advocate regulation as a solution. Basically, the regulatory approach leaves the technologies intact while making them less haphazard. It restricts the more egregious abuses of these technologies by legislating the conditions and the contexts in which they can be used and by watchdogging the ways in which these technologies are abused, for example, when a woman is given Norplant without her consent. Regulation functions as quality control rather than as critical challenge.

Regulation is a perceived rational response advocating restriction rather than abolition, and within the dominant medical and commercial ecology of reproductive technologies and contracts, scientists, lawyers, and entrepreneurs have made a plea for this kind of legislation.

Regulation is exactly what the supporters and developers of technological reproduction want. It gives the surrogate brokers, for example, a stable marketing environment and makes the process of surrogacy more convenient for the client and broker. It also gives the IVF clinics a way of quality-controlling their success rates so that only the most successful centers survive and the competition is edged out. Regulation thus amounts to self-regulation as, for example, in the American Fertility Association's report on new reproductive procedures.

The regulatory approach is also based on a sense of the inevitability of the new reproductive technologies. The message is that it is useless to prevent such procedures since they have already gained prevailing ground; that many women want and need them; and that prohibition will drive them underground. Even if outlawing surrogacy, for example, did drive it underground, the number of surrogate arrangements would be minuscule compared to the explosive growth of surrogacy that would result from permissive regulation. Yet this sense of inevitability has given way to a perception of legal necessity leading to continued use and legitimation of new reproductive procedures. *Is* becomes *ought*. Caution rather than resistance becomes the norm. Regulation encourages adaptation rather than a search for alternatives or an outright rejection of a technology.

In the United States, there has always been more of an institutional momentum for regulation than abolition. Part of this momentum can be attributed to the value that Americans place on choice and laissez-faire individualism, but it is also bound up with the perception that to prohibit any of these new reproductive procedures is technological McCarthyism—a repressive, retrogressive censorship of progress and a gross intrusion into the reproductive lives of individuals who may need the techniques.

In the case of surrogacy, many state legislatures have crafted or are in the process of considering regulatory legislation that will get rid of the grosser inequities of the surrogate contract. Some of these regulatory bills allow the so-called surrogate to change her mind after the child is born, but only if she is willing to contest her claim in court and most likely to endure a custody battle. Thus she must hire a lawyer and have the financial wherewithal to challenge the greater legal and financial advantages of the sperm source. Other bills restrict any money from changing hands as a payment for reproductive services but allow money to be exchanged for "necessary expenses" or as a gift. Thus these very limits, enacted supposedly to protect the surrogate, do not provide her with the concrete *means* of protection from abuse that are available only to the powerful, that is, to the sperm source or the contracting couple or the brokerage agency.

Regulatory surrogacy legislation has tightened up not only the contract, but also the supervision and regulation of the woman's behavior while pregnant. As in legalized prostitution where the state becomes the brothel, so too in legalized surrogacy the state becomes the broker. "The regulations governing prostitution (medical check-ups, cards and brothels) were historically one of the main causes of the prostitution of women, and still are, because they do not allow them to abandon this activity and return to their social group. Because of the regulations, they come to form a separate category of women living on the fringes of society, who are vulnerable and 'marked for life.'"[22] Likewise, regulatory surrogacy legislation brands a certain class of women as surrogate breeders. Laws that claim to regulate surrogacy end up promoting it.

Finally, regulation saves women from perhaps some of the more abusive aspects of the new reproductive technologies, but as a private privilege, not as a political human right. It provides no public protection for women, as women, against medical invasions of bodily integrity; it fails to prevent a new version of reproductive servitude from taking root as reproductive choice; and it encourages the exporting of surrogacy to countries where women's bodies are cheaper and there are no regulations.

If we take seriously the right of women to bodily integrity, we must also urge the passage of legislation against the new reproductive procedures that is premised on a more substantive right to personal and political integrity. Such legislation must address not merely the effects of technological reproduction but the causes as well and must acknowledge the violation of a woman's bodily integrity. "Feminists who think regulation would protect the mother miss the whole point of the maternity contract, which is precisely to deprive her of the protections she would have if she had signed nothing."[23]

In examining environmental legislation in the United States, H. Patricia Hynes asks the question whether more environmental laws guarantee more environmental protection. The Federal Insecticide, Fungicide, and Rodenticide Act (FIFRA) gave EPA the right to review all new pesticides before they could be sold and used and to review all new uses for old pesticides. In looking at the way in which FIFRA was enforced, however, Hynes found the law gave only the appearance and language of protection but not necessarily the reality of it. Because the intentionality of the law was to register chemicals and their uses, to close the more glaring loopholes that environmental activists of the 1960s had identified, and to keep chemicals on the market without letting them run rampant in agriculture, "it placed a mantle of protection around the use of chemical pesticides."[24]

Citing FIFRA's lack of ecological intentionality, Hynes contends that the law could have been written to promote a sustainable agriculture without chemicals that maximized, instead, the use of organic farming, biological controls, and integrated pest management (IPM). It could have contained no loophole allowing the manufacture or sale of chemicals banned in the United States in other, particularly Third World, countries. A law that had ecological intentionality "would intend to protect people and global ecology, not the chemical market. It would be a law intent on 'risk elimination, reduction, and minimization,' not risk management. This is what I mean by intentionality."[25]

Regulations that place only certain limits on contractual and technological reproduction lack a similar intentionality. This kind of regulatory legislation intends only to manage the risks to women, not to eliminate those risks. And, as we have seen with other reproductive drugs such as Depo-Provera, when a treatment or technology is banned for use in the United States, it is often exported to women in developing countries.

Ultimately, in this book I contend that the best legal approach to reproductive technologies and contracts that violate women's bodily integrity—such as IVF and its offshoots, egg donation, sex predetermination, fetal reduction, fetal tissue use for research and transplants, surrogacy, sterilization abuse, and invasive injectable and implantable contraception of Third World women—is abolition, not regulation. The starting point for the protection of women's bodily integrity is the abolition of technological reproduction by penalizing its vendors and purveyors and by preventing women from being technologically ravaged.

Before legislation, however, we must strengthen feminist action and activism at all levels. Action has to be the foundation and base for any legislation that is gender specific and international. Technological reproduction is a transnational, as well as a national, traffic in women that is promoted by organized medicine, marketing, and media. Any interventions at the national level must also be enforced internationally, and any laws enacted must not limit women's rights in other areas of female existence.

As one concrete example, women need an International Convention against medical exploitation developed by governmental and nongovernmental organizations (NGOs) that would declare women's right to bodily integrity, support women's established right to human dignity and physical well-being, and work to prohibit the expansionism of contractual and technological reproduction. Perhaps set in a larger context of medical violations of women's human rights, such a convention would specifically recognize contractual and technological reproduction as a violation of women's human rights, addressing its role in promoting an international reproductive traffic in women, and making clear that it constitutes a severe form of sexual and reproductive exploitation.

No radical feminist believes that legislation itself will bring an end to women's sexual and reproductive subordination. Legislation can often be subverted for male-dominant purposes, but regulatory legislation makes that subversion all the more likely. Regulatory legislation encourages reams of rules and restrictions having the potential to generate legal conflicts that end up in layer upon layer of litigation. It is easy to imagine an accretion of reforms in relation to surrogacy, for instance, that, instead of effecting transformation of the conditions that draw women into surrogacy, further normalizes, rationalizes, and institutionalizes reproductive servitude. Regulatory legislation manages rather than stops the traffic in women and children, like a blinking traffic light that slows traffic, but only at certain points, and then allows it to start up again at its normal pace. A radical feminist politics takes seriously the need to provide women with a full stop to this battle over women's bodies. A radical feminist politics demands technological justice.

Introduction

1. See Robyn Rowland, *Living Laboratories* (Bloomington: Indiana Univ. Press, 1992).
2. See Robert Jay Lifton, *The Nazi Doctors: Medical Killing and the Psychology of Genocide* (New York: Basic Books, 1986), 472, for a delineation of totalistic ideology.
3. Erwin Chargaff, "Engineering a Molecular Nightmare," *Nature* 327 (1987): 199–200.
4. Calvin Miller, "IVF 'Out of Control' as European Embryo Stockpiles Grow," *The Herald*, January 23, 1989.
5. Laparoscopic egg collection is used during IVF to remove a woman's eggs by inserting a laparoscope (light guide), a suction device, and forceps to grasp a woman's ovary. A woman undergoing laparoscopic egg collection must submit to abdominal incision, general anesthesia, and inflation of the abdomen with carbon dioxide gas.
6. Gail Batman, ed., *In-Vitro Fertilisation in Australia* (Canberra, Australia: Commonwealth Department of Community Services and Health, 1988).
7. Superovulation is a procedure used by fertility specialists to induce a woman to produce large numbers of eggs instead of the usual one that is generated during monthly ovulation. Clinicians use powerful fertility drugs to coax the ovaries into yielding multiple eggs, frequently resulting in overstimulation and enlargement of a woman's ovaries with the danger of rupture.

8. Anita Goldman, "The Production of Eggs," in *Infertility: Women Speak Out About Their Experiences of Reproductive Medicine*, ed. Renate Klein (London: Pandora, 1989), 70.

9. Goldman, "Production of Eggs," 71.

10. Gena Corea, *The Zenaide Project*, Work-in-Progress on the Deaths of Women Resulting from IVF Treatment, Institute on Women and Technology, Box 338, N. Amherst, Massachusetts 01059; see also Ana Regina Gomes Dos Reis, "IVF in Brazil: The Story Told by the Newspapers," in *Made to Order: The Myth of Reproductive and Genetic Progress*, ed. P. Spallone and D. Steinberg (New York: Pergamon, 1987), 120–32; see again, Alison Solomon, "Sometimes Pergonal Kills," in *Infertility*, ed. Klein, 46–50; and finally, see the various accounts of Denise Mounce's death in, for example, Ena Naunton, "The Untimely Death of a Surrogate Mother," *The Miami Herald*, May 1, 1988. Denise's mother, Pat Mounce, has testified tirelessly at both state and congressional hearings against surrogacy legislation that would make the contracts legal and enforceable, as well as against any bills that would regulate surrogate contracts. She has often stated, "I have a very *personal* interest in supporting legislation which would put the baby brokers out of business." Denise Mounce had a developmental abnormality of the heart wherein she suffered rapid heartbeat. Medical records show that the broker's obstetrician knew about this condition, at least when the pregnancy was under way, and that the broker also knew. The former referred her to a cardiologist who told her to return with 250 dollars to be fitted with a halter heart monitor. She had no money so she never went back, and about one month later, she died of acute heart failure. The fetus also died.

11. Susan Sontag, *Illness as Metaphor* (New York: Vintage Books, 1979), 81.

12. Office of Technology Assessment (OTA), *Infertility: Medical and Social Choices*, Office of Technology Report, U.S. Congress, May 1988.

13. "Test-Tube Kids Bred at Rye," *Southern Peninsula Gazette*, February 17, 1988.

14. Bill Handel, quoted in Gena Corea, *The Mother Machine: Reproductive Technologies from Artificial Insemination to Artificial Wombs* (New York: Harper & Row, 1985), 217.

15. See Rebecca Powers and Sheila Gruber Belloli, "Another Surrogacy Arranged Through Noel Keane Goes Awry," *The Detroit News*, January 14, 1991, 7B. Kathleen King, another of Noel Keane's hired contract mothers, stated that she underwent the psychological screening required by the agency and, when she was not approved, was asked to sign a waiver acknowledging she had failed but in spite of this would comply with the contract.

16. See Gena Corea and Susan Ince, "IVF a Game for Losers at Half of U.S. Clinics," *Medical Tribune* 26 (19) (July 3, 1985): 1, 12–13. Reprinted as

"Report of a Survey of IVF Clinics in the US," in *Made to Order: The Myth of Reproductive and Genetic Progress,* ed. Spallone (New York: Pergamon, 1987), esp. 133–39.

17. *Matter of Baby M.*, 525 A.2d 1128, 1166 (NJ Super. Ct. Ch. Div. 1987), rev'd, 537 A.2d 1127 (NJ 1988).

18. Patrick Steptoe at a "Women, Reproduction and Technology" Conference, the History Workshop Centre, Oxford, February 14–15, 1987, quoted in Michelle Stanworth, ed., *Reproductive Technologies* (London: Polity Press, 1987), 15.

19. H. Patricia Hynes, *The Recurring Silent Spring* (New York: Pergamon, 1989), 8.

20. United Nations Economic and Social Council, "Contemporary Forms of Slavery," *Report of the Working Group on Contemporary Forms of Slavery on Its Sixteenth Session,* Mrs. F. Z. Ksentini, Rapporteur, Commission on Human Rights, Sub-Commission on Prevention of Discrimination and Protection of Minorities, Geneva, Switzerland, July 1991, 1–53.

21. Interview with John Stehura, president of the Bionetics Foundation, a reproductive services and surrogate agency, quoted in Gena Corea, *The Mother Machine* (New York: Harper & Row, 1985), 214–15. Stehura specifically suggested Central America.

22. Raised by several delegates to the CEDAW (Committee on the Elimination of Discrimination Against Women) meetings at the United Nations and part of the public record of these meetings. See reports of the State Parties and minutes of the Eleventh Session of the Committee on the Elimination of Discrimination Against Women, January 20–31, 1992.

23. Piet Stoffelen, Rapporteur, *Parliamentary Assembly Report on the Traffic in Children and Other Forms of Child Exploitation,* Council of Europe, September 10, 1987, 1–16. This report is based on the findings of Interpol, the Anti-Slavery Society, the International Labour Organization, various UN groups, adoption agencies, and local newspaper reports.

24. Vibuti Patel, "Sex-Determination and Sex Preselection Tests in India: Recent Techniques in Femicide," *Reproductive and Genetic Engineering* 2, no. 2 (1989): 111–19. Patel refers in this article to several investigative reports that unearthed these figures in popular magazines such as *India Today* and the *Times of India.*

25. *Nature* 324 (November 20, 1986): 202.

26. Patel, "Sex-Determination and Sex Preselection," 114.

27. Mary O'Brien, *The Politics of Reproduction* (Boston: Routledge & Kegan Paul, 1981), 8.

28. G. J. Barker-Benfield, *The Horrors of the Half-Known Life: Male Attitudes Toward Women and Sexuality in Nineteenth-Century America* (New York: Harper & Row, 1976); see especially chapter 15, "The Spermatic Economy and Proto-Sublimation."

29. Diana Scully, *Men Who Control Women's Health: The Education of Obstetricians and Gynecologists* (New York: Houghton Mifflin, 1980).

30. Anne Marie Moulin, review of *L'oeuf transparent,* by Jacques Testart, *Journal of Medicine and Philosophy* 14 (1989): 587–91.

31. Jacques Testart, quoted in Somer Brodribb, *Women and Reproductive Technologies,* Background Study Report Prepared for the Status of Women in Canada, May 20, 1988, 33–34.

32. Brigitte Oberauer, "Baby Making in Austria," in *Infertility,* ed. Klein, 114.

33. Quoted in Gena Corea, "Surrogacy: Making the Links," in *Infertility,* ed. Klein, 135.

34. Elizabeth Kane, *Birth Mother: The Story of America's First Legal Surrogate Mother* (New York: Harcourt Brace Jovanovich, 1988), 81.

35. Jalna Hanmer, "Transforming Consciousness: Women and the New Reproductive Technologies," in Gena Corea et al., *Man-Made Women: How the New Reproductive Technologies Affect Women* (Bloomington and Indianapolis: Indiana Univ. Press, 1987), 106.

36. Powers and Gruber Belloli, "Another Surrogacy," 7B.

37. Louise Vandelac, "Mothergate: Surrogate Mothers, Linguistics, and Androcentric Engineering," trans. Jane Parniak and Lise Moisan, *Resources for Feminist Research/Documentation sur la recherche féministe* 15, no. 4 (1987): 41–47.

38. Elizabeth Kane, Unpublished lecture given at the National Women's Studies Association Meeting (NWSA), University of Minnesota, June 24, 1988, 4.

39. Quoted in Kane, *Birth Mother,* 74.

40. Brigitte Oberauer, "Baby Making in Austria," in *Infertility,* ed. Klein, 113.

41. Renate Klein, *The Exploitation of a Desire: Women's Experiences with In Vitro Fertilization* (Geelong, Victoria, Australia: Deakin Univ. Press, 1989), 31.

42. Margaret Jackson, "*The Political* versus *The Natural*: Case Studies in the Struggle for Female Sexual Autonomy (1800–1940)" (Ph.D. diss., Univ. of Birmingham, England, 1990), 431.

43. Jacques Testart, on introducing the performance to the audience, at the inaugural ceremonies of the Seventh World Congress on In Vitro Fertilization and Assisted Procreations, Paris, June 30, 1991.

Chapter 1. The Production of Fertility and Infertility: East and West, South and North

1. Vimal Balasubrahmanyan, "Women as Targets in India's Family Planning Policy," in *Test-Tube Women: What Future for Motherhood?* ed. Rita Arditti, Renate Duelli Klein, and Shelley Minden (Boston: Pandora, 1984), 153–64. The author correlates the political defeat of Indira Gandhi and her Congress Party in 1977 with the increased pressures put on women to undergo sterilization. "Feminists in India feel that this policy shift is based

on the belief that women, whatever be the FP [Family Planning] onslaughts on them, will not express their displeasure through the ballot box. The . . . vasectomy compulsions did result in decisive votes *against* the Congress government" (155).

2. Many women who undergo IVF have already endured many infertility treatments and workups that are extremely painful and physically intrusive. Many are also infertile due to the ravages of harmful contraception and sexually transmitted disease.

3. Office of Technology Assessment, "Infertility: Medical and Social Choices," OTA Report Brief, May 1988 (Washington, DC: Government Printing Office), stock no. 052-003-01091-7.

4. Between 25 and 60 percent of couples who are infertile and who seek help from fertility clinics will have a child in the traditional heterosexual way, that is, without any assistance from any kind of treatment. See Louise Vandelac with the collaboration of Maria De Koninck, "From Reproductive Technologies to the Industrialization of Life," trans. Lucille Nelson, in *Reproductive Technologies and Women: A Research Tool/Femmes et technologies de procréation: Outils de Recherches*, ed. CRIAW/ICREF Working Group on Reproductive Technologies (Ottawa, Ontario: CRIAW/ICREF, 1989), 20; in the French, 77–91.

5. All information and statistics are from William Mosher and William Pratt, "Fecundity and Infertility in the United States, 1965–82," in NCHS *Advancedata*, from Vital and Health Statistics of the National Center of Health Statistics, U.S. Dept. of Health and Human Services no. 104 (February 11, 1985).

6. *Time* magazine used this phrase most recently in its cover story, "Making Babies," September 30, 1991, written by Philip Elmer-Dewitt. Although the story quoted the correct statistic of one in twelve couples having difficulty in conceiving, it nevertheless conveyed the impression that this was a recent statistic of expanding proportions rather than an infertility rate that has remained consistent since 1965.

7. OTA Report Brief, "Infertility: Medical and Social Choices."

8. *Matter of Baby M.*, 525 A.2d 1128, 1161 (NJ Super. Ct. Ch. Div. 1987), rev'd, 537 A.2d 1227 (NJ 1988).

9. *Matter of Baby M.*

10. Rochelle A. Stackhouse, Letter to the Editor, *Ms. Magazine*, August 1988, 12.

11. See Ute Winkler and Traute Schonenberg, "Options for Involuntarily Childless Women," in *Infertility: Women Speak Out About Their Experiences of Reproductive Medicine*, ed. Renate Klein (London: Pandora, 1989), 207–24.

12. Quoted in Jane Fraser, "Putting Male Infertility Under the Microscope," *The Australian*, March 4, 1987, 10.

13. Fraser, "Male Infertility," 10.

14. The "In Vitro Fertilization-Embryo Transfer (IVF-ET) in the United States: 1989 Results from the IVF-ET Registry" states that 28 percent of the total number of transfer cycles undertaken using GIFT (Gamete Intrafallopian Transfer) were done because of the infertility diagnosis of "male factor"; 23 percent of the total number of stimulation cycles undertaken using IVF were done because of the infertility diagnosis of "male factor." See the report in *Fertility and Sterility* 55, no. 1 (January 1991). These figures may well be conservative statistics since the registry is an in-house report of the American Fertility Society supported by a contract from Serono Laboratories, the maker of the fertility drug Pergonal. Indeed, according to Dr. Georgeanna Seegar Jones and Dr. Howard Jones, Jr., founders of the Jones Institute for Reproductive Medicine at the Eastern Virginia Medical School in Norfolk, Virginia, it is the male who has the fertility problem in 60 percent of the couples seeking help. The latter figure of 60 percent was quoted in Sue Miller, "More Older Women Decide to Try In Vitro Fertilization," *Eugene Register Guard*, June 18, 1989.

15. John Elkington, *The Age*, July 8, 1985, 15.

16. Dr. David Bradford, a specialist in sexually transmitted diseases, quoted in Philip McIntosh, "Is In Vitro the Real Answer to Infertility?" *The Age*, July 26, 1985.

17. Vandelac with De Konick, "Reproductive Technologies," 19.

18. Quoted in "Going for Gold in the Baby Business," *Fortune*, September 17, 1984, 33–36. Exclamation point mine.

19. A total of 224 clinics nationwide were cited in the congressional study entitled "Consumer Protection Issues Involving In Vitro Fertilization Clinics," U.S. House of Representatives Subcommittee on Regulation, Business and Energy, March 1989, 100 pages. Available from the U.S. House of Representatives Subcommittee on Regulation, Business and Energy, Committee on Small Business, R-363, Rayburn House Office Building, Washington, DC 20515.

20. "Consumer Protection Issues." Other studies cite from 6,000 to 8,000 dollars per cycle.

21. Many magazine and newspaper articles carried reports about the debate in Australia over the marketing of IVF technology abroad. The passage of the Infertility (Medical Procedures) Act in 1984 made the commercialization of IVF technology impossible in Victoria. IVF Australia was initially an attempt to realize a profit abroad, using publicly funded research, done in Australia, for private profit gained outside the country. See, for example, Glennys Bell, "How Australia's Unique Techniques Are Being Exported," *The Bulletin*, July 16, 1985, 70–75. In the United States, IVF Australia's—now IVF America's—advertisements are carried in major newspapers, for example, in a full-page ad in the *New York Times Magazine*, April 17, 1988.

22. Alison Leigh Cowan, "Can a Baby-Making Venture Deliver?" *The New York Times,* June 1, 1992, D1.

23. Cowan, "Baby-Making Venture," D1.

24. Cowan, "Baby-Making Venture," D6.

25. American Fertility Society, "In Vitro Fertilization-Embryo Transfer (IVF-ET) in the United States: 1989 Results from the IVF-ET Registry," *Fertility and Sterility* 55, no. 1 (January 1991): 23.

26. Quoted in International Medical News Service, "High-Tech Infertility Treatments Offer Some Remedy for Almost Every Fertility Problem," *Ob. Gyn. News* 19, no. 24 (December 15, 1984): 1.

27. Quoted in Gena Corea and Susan Ince, "IVF a Game for Losers at Half of U.S. Clinics," *Medical Tribune* 26, no. 19 (July 3, 1985): 12. Reprinted as "Report of a Survey of IVF Clinics in the USA," in *Made to Order: The Myth of Reproductive and Genetic Progress,* ed. Patricia Spallone and Deborah Lynn Steinberg (New York: Pergamon, 1987), 135.

28. Quoted in Gena Corea, *The Mother Machine: Reproductive Technologies from Artificial Insemination to Artificial Wombs* (New York: Harper & Row, 1985), 179.

29. Renate Klein, "Resistance: From the Exploitation of Infertility to an Exploration of In-Fertility," in *Infertility,* ed. Klein, 233.

30. It is important to note that at the point that some women advance to the egg recovery stage, many other women have been turned away from the IVF programs, having been judged as bad candidates for egg harvesting. These "bad candidates" have gone through the first stages of IVF tests and treatment, however, but are not counted in the statistics. Instead, they are categorized as "canceled" cycles and thus not specified as IVF treatment failures but as women whose eggs are not suitable or cannot be harvested. One U.S. study estimates that the number of these "canceled" cycles is substantial, as high as 41.6 percent of all women who begin IVF programs. See Sung I. Roh et al., "In Vitro Fertilization and Embryo Transfer: Treatment-Dependent versus Independent Pregnancies," *Fertility and Sterility,* 48, no. 6 (December 1987): 982–86.

31. Office of Technology Assessment, "Infertility: Medical and Social Choices" (Washington, DC: GPO, 1988), stock no. 052-003-01091-7.

32. U.S. House of Representatives Subcommittee on Regulation, Business and Energy, 1989 study. The Wyden statistics were discussed in Miriam Tucker, "Congress Eyes Possibility of Regulating Infertility Clinics: Releases Results of Success Rate Survey," *Ob. Gyn. News* 24, no. 8 (April 15–30, 1989): 1, 42.

33. Voluntary Licensing Authority for Human In Vitro Fertilization and Embryology, *Third Report* (London, 1988); FIVNAT Report (France, 1987); Gail Batman, *In-Vitro Fertilisation in Australia,* Commonwealth Department of Community Services and Health (Canberra, Australia, 1988). Statistics reported in Australia were from 1986 and 1987.

34. National Perinatal Statistics Unit and the Fertility Society of Australia, "In Vitro Fertilization Pregnancies, Australia and New Zealand, 1979–85," National Perinatal Statistics Unit (Sydney, 1987), 2, 8–13. The national IVF register examines all IVF pregnancies in Australia and New Zealand. This was the third report in a series based on the register of IVF births in both countries. The first was published in 1984.

35. See a further report on "Congenital Malformations after In-Vitro Fertilisation," by Paul A. L. Lancaster, National Perinatal Statistics Unit, *The Lancet* vol. II for 1987 (December 12, 1987), no. 8275, 1392.

36. VLA (Voluntary Licensing Authority) for Human In Vitro Fertilization and Embryology, *Third Report* (London, 1988). An abridged summary of this report appeared in "Sale of Human Eggs Should Be Outlawed," *New Scientist*, May 27, 1989, 31. The VLA is a voluntary watchdog group set up by members supportive of the development of these reproductive technologies.

37. National Perinatal Statistics Unit and the Fertility Society of Australia, "In Vitro Fertilization Pregnancies."

38. National Perinatal Statistics Unit.

39. "Reassuring Study on In Vitro Babies," *New York Times*, August 11, 1989, A17.

40. Richard Saltus, "Study Dispels Fears of High Rate of Birth Defects in 'Test-tube' Babies," *Boston Globe*, August 10, 1989, 9.

41. GIFT stands for gamete intrafallopian transfer, a variation of IVF in which eggs harvested from a woman and sperm taken from her partner or a donor are injected into the woman's fallopian tube to enable fertilization to occur there instead of in the petri dish, the usual IVF method of fertilization. Doctors believe that, with some women, GIFT has a higher success rate and is more "natural." ZIFT is yet another variation of GIFT in which the fertilized egg (zygote) is transferred into the fallopian tube. TUDOR is the acronym for transvaginal ultrasound-directed oocyte (egg) recovery, a technique used to collect eggs through the vagina instead of via laparoscopy, a surgical method of egg harvesting.

42. It is important to understand that IVF is not one procedure alone but, for women, involves several steps: superovulation with powerful fertility drugs to force the production of multiple eggs; laparoscopy or ultrasound-directed egg retrieval to harvest these eggs; fertilization of the eggs with sperm, either outside the woman's body in a laboratory (petri) dish or inside the fallopian tube; and often the implanting of multiple embryos into the woman's body. If several embryos "take," doctors frequently perform a fetal reduction procedure to terminate some embryos in utero.

43. The doctor was removed from the suit because he would not agree to the settlement. Although he was confident a jury would vindicate him, nonetheless his insurance company was unwilling to take that risk. See Nancy

Hill-Holtzman, "Frustacis Settle Suit over Birth of Septuplets," *Los Angeles Times*, April 29, 1990, A1. In a bizarre twist, however, Patti Frustaci underwent further fertility treatment with the same drug, Pergonal, at another clinic in southern California and in January 1991 gave birth to twins. The Frustacis had charged in their lawsuit that the clinic and the doctor had neglected to order ultrasound to determine the number of egg receptacles present in Patti Frustaci before insemination. The doctor claimed Patti Frustaci had refused the test. See *New York Times*, "Twins for Mother of Septuplets," January 24, 1991.

44. A 1992 study in the *American Journal of Epidemiology* reported that women who took fertility drugs were three times more likely to experience ovarian cancer than women who never took the drugs. And, if these women did not become pregnant after superovulation, the risk of ovarian cancer was 27 times higher. The study, led by Stanford University epidemiologist Alice Whittemore, documented these risks based on a review of 12 previous ovarian cancer studies involving over 11,000 women. Alice S. Whittemore et al., "Characteristics Relating to Ovarian Cancer Risk: Collaborative Analysis of 12 U.S. Case-Control Studies I–IV," *American Journal of Epidemiology* 136, 10 (November 15, 1992): 1175–1220.

45. Rose Gutfeld, "FDA Says Labels of Fertility Drugs Must Warn Users," *Wall Street Journal*, January 14, 1993, B6.

46. Renate Klein and Robyn Rowland, "Women as Test-Sites for Fertility Drugs," *Reproductive and Genetic Engineering* 1, no. 3 (1988): 251–73.

47. UNESCO, International Symposium on the Effects on Human Rights of Recent Advances in Science and Technology. Organized by the International Social Science Council, Conclusions and Recommendations (Paris: Division of Human Rights, 1985), publication SHS-86/QA/39.

48. Christa Wichterich, "From the Struggle Against 'Overpopulation' to the Industrialization of Human Production," *Reproductive and Genetic Engineering* 1, no. 1 (1988): 25.

49. Morton Mintz, *At Any Cost: Corporate Greed, Women, and the Dalkon Shield* (New York: Pantheon, 1985), 4–6. Mintz reports that Dalkon Shield insertions were carried out in African, Asian, Middle Eastern, Caribbean, Latin American, and South American countries in which poor medical conditions made lethal complications more likely. "My guess is that Shield-related PID killed hundreds—possibly thousands—of women outside of the United States" (4). After the sales of the shield were suspended in the United States, the lawyer for many U.S. women who had been harmed by the device asked A. H. Robins, chairman, why the company had collected all unsold shields from the market in the United States. "Because it was the proper thing to do," said Chairman Robins. If it was the "proper thing to do," the lawyer asked Robins, why wasn't the "proper thing" also done for women in the developing countries? "To all such questions the chairman's

answer was that he did not know" (5). Mintz reports that after halting domestic sales, A. H. Robins continued to distribute shields abroad for nine months. One family planning worker in El Salvador recalled that clinics in El Salvador continued to implant shields until 1980 (5).

The Dalkon Shield story is an outrageous and tragic story of social injustice, medical mutilation, and death for thousands of women. For a rigorous, inspiring, and remarkable study of how many Dalkon Shield survivors in the United States empowered themselves, see Karen M. Hicks, *Surviving the Dalkon Shield IUD: Women v. the Pharmaceutical Industry* (New York: Teachers College Press, 1993).

50. Multicenter testing of the type sponsored by the World Health Organization is done in many countries, at one time, often with a majority of test sites in developing countries.

51. The Population Council is a nonprofit research center based in New York that has a history of researching and developing population control methods. The 4 percent profits figure was reported by Philip J. Hilts, "U.S. Approves 5-Year Implants to Curb Fertility," *New York Times*, December 11, 1990, B10.

52. Ana Regina Gomes Dos Reis, "Norplant in Brazil: Implantation Strategy in the Guise of Scientific Research," *Reproductive and Genetic Engineering* 3, no. 2 (1990): 111–18.

53. Ana Regina Gomes Dos Reis makes the important point that behind the term *increased bleeding* are hidden blood losses that would be considered pathological if the classic gynecological terms and concepts, such as menorrhea and hypermenorrhea, were used. Interviews with Norplant users taped by feminist groups reveal that many women had continuous bleeding lasting for twenty or even thirty days. The impact of these so-called irregularities on these women's day-to-day life and health was ignored. When the women complained about the excessive bleeding, they were informed that this was "normal" and that if they waited the symptoms would eventually disappear. The change in menstruation is, however, the main cause for removal of the implants, which demonstrates that this is not a "normal" biological behavioral pattern for women (114–15).

54. UBINIG, "Research Report: Norplant, the Five Year Needle: An Investigation of the Norplant Trial in Bangladesh from the User's Perspective," *Reproductive and Genetic Engineering* 3, no. 3 (1990): 212. This promotion continued despite the fact that Wayne Bardin, vice president of the Population Council and director of its Centre for Biomedical Research, acknowledged that sterilization failure is 1 percent per thousand, and Norplant failure is 3 percent per thousand.

55. UBINIG, "Norplant," 213.

56. UBINIG, "Norplant," 214.

57. UBINIG, "Norplant," 219.

58. UBINIG, "Norplant," 220.

59. UBINIG, "Norplant," 227.

60. Farida Akhter, "Report on the FINRRAGE-UBINIG Regional Meeting, Held at BARD, Comilla, May 8–11, 1990," *Reproductive and Genetic Engineering* 3, no. 3 (1990): 297–99.

61. Draft statement on Norplant, Anti-Pregnancy Vaccines, and RU 486 Presented at the Sixth International Women's Health Meeting, November 3–9, 1990, Quezon City, Philippines.

62. Reported in "Mabuhay! The International Women's Health Movement is Alive and Well," *ISIS* Women's Health Journal 20 (October–December 1990): 12.

63. Quoted in Jo Salomone, "Report on the 6th International Women and Health Meeting, November 3–9, 1990, Manila, Philippines," *Issues in Reproductive and Genetic Engineering: Journal of International Feminist Analysis* 4, no. 1 (1991): 82.

64. "Showdown over Quality: Planners Face Up to Feminists in Family Planning Conference," *ISIS* Women's Health Journal 19 (July–September 1990): 64.

65. "Showdown Over Quality," 65.

66. See Janice G. Raymond, Renate Klein, and Lynette Dumble, *RU 486: Misconceptions, Myths, and Morals* (Cambridge: Institute on Women and Technology, MIT, 1991; and North Melbourne, Victoria: Spinfex Press, 1991).

67. Clare Booth Luce, "Fewer Moms Would Slow the Pop Clock," *The Seattle Times,* August 6, 1978, K6.

68. John Postgate, "Bat's Chance in Hell," *New Scientist,* April 5, 1973, 14.

69. Paul Ehrlich, *The Population Bomb,* rev. ed. (New York: Ballantine, 1971), 133.

70. Vibuti Patel, "Campaign Against Amniocentesis," in *In Search of Our Bodies: A Feminist Look at Women, Health, and Reproduction in India,* ed. Kamakshi Bhate et al. (Bombay: Shakti Publishing, 1987), 70–74.

71. Quoted in Lakshmi Lingam, "Reproductive Technologies in India," *Issues in Reproductive and Genetic Engineering* 3, no. 1 (1990): 15, emphasis mine.

72. PIVET Australia (from Programmed In Vitro Fertilisation and Embryo Transfer), based in Perth, is the biggest privately owned IVF team in Australia. "A stream of overseas scientists tread a path to its door intent on returning home and establishing infertility clinics," reports the *Bulletin* of Monash University (June 19, 1986). Who is treading a path to whose door is, of course, a debatable question with PIVET establishing laboratory, research, and clinical complexes in many areas of the world.

73. Sex predetermination methods have been emphasized by governmental representatives and some so-called intellectuals as the best means to lower

the birth rate to 2.3, the goal of the Sixth and Seventh Five-Year Plan, documents that target net reproductive rates. Lingam, "Reproductive Technologies," 20.

74. In 1901, for example, there were 972 Indian women per 1,000 men. By comparison with India's current rate of 920 women per 1,000 men, the United States has 105 women for every 100 men, which is the norm in the developed countries.

75. Barbara Crossette, "India's Population Put at 844 Million," *New York Times*, March 26, 1991, A6.

76. Crossette, "India's Population," A6.

77. Irene Sege, "The Grim Mystery of World's Missing Women," *Boston Globe*, February 3, 1992, 23.

78. See Nancy E. Williamson, "Boys or Girls? Parents' Preferences and Sex Control," *Population Bulletin* 33, no. 1 (January 1978), for a survey of evidence from the United States and selected countries on what types of preferences parents have about the sexes of their children and how strongly they are held. See also Helen G. Holmes, Betty B. Hoskins, and Michael Gross, *The Custom-Made Child?* (Clinton, NJ: Humana Press, 1981); see especially the section on "Sex Preselection" organized by Janice G. Raymond, 177–224.

79. Vibuti Patel, "Sex Determination and Preselection Tests in India: Recent Techniques in Femicide," *Reproductive and Genetic Engineering* 2, no. 2 (1989): 113.

80. Dr. Jaswant Singh, who teaches at the Rohtak Medical College, has stated, "We know of many cases where the woman was not keen on this test, but their family pressured them." Quoted in Edward Gargan, "Ultrasound Skews India's Birth Ratio," *New York Times*, December 13, 1991, A13.

81. Dr. Hema Purandare, quoted in Bharathsadasivam, "The Silent Scream," *Illustrated Weekly of India*, September 14, 1986, 40.

82. Patel, "Sex Determination and Preselection Tests," 115.

83. Amanda LeGrand, "Medical and Users' Aspects of RU 486 with Particular Emphasis on Its Use in Third World Countries," in WEMOS, *Women and Pharmaceuticals Proceedings on RU 486, the Abortion Pill* (Amsterdam, 1990).

84. Vibuti Patel, quoted in Kirsten Ellis and Seema Sirohi, *The Australian*, May 18, 1987.

85. Patel, "Sex Determination and Preselection Tests," 117.

86. Ann Pappert, "A Voice for Infertile Women," in *Infertility*, ed. Klein, 198.

87. Pappert, "A Voice for Infertile Women," 204.

88. Pappert, "A Voice for Infertile Women," 204.

89. H. Patricia Hynes, *The Recurring Silent Spring* (New York: Pergamon, 1989), 17.

Chapter 2. Maternal Environments and Ejaculatory Fathers:
New Definitions of Motherhood and Fatherhood

1. Somer Brodribb, "ReproTech: Script for a New Generation," *Broadside* 10, no. 5 (1989): 11.
2. I use the term *essentialism* throughout this work in the following ways: the theory that certain attributes, qualities, and functions define a group or class and/or belong to them by nature—of their essence; the properties by means of which something can be placed in its proper class or identified as being what it is; something that is inherent, basic, indispensable, or necessary to a group's being.
3. Thirty-eight expert and lay witnesses testified in the initial New Jersey Superior Court Trial in 1987, and their "findings" about Mary Beth Whitehead's fitness for motherhood are referred to throughout this legal decision: *Matter of Baby M.*, 525 A.2d 1128 (NJ Super. Ct. Ch. Div. 1987), rev'd, 537 A.2d 1227 (NJ 1988).
4. *Matter of Baby M.*, at 1170, 1168, 1169.
5. *Matter of Baby M.*, at 1139.
6. *Matter of Baby M.*, at 1157, emphasis added.
7. *Matter of Baby M.*, at 1169, emphasis added.
8. This theme runs throughout Simone de Beauvoir, *The Second Sex*, trans. and ed. H. M. Parshley (New York: Bantam, 1952).
9. *Matter of Baby M.*, at 1157, 1227.
10. Judith Levine, "Motherhood Is Powerless," *Village Voice*, April 14, 1987, 15–16.
11. It is perhaps not widely known that within the last decade especially, fathers are fighting and winning child custody battles at an astounding rate. Phyllis Chesler's study, *Mothers on Trial: The Battle for Children and Custody* (New York: Harcourt Brace Jovanovich, 1991), not only summarizes the current studies to date, which document the results of custody disputes, but uses original work on a representative sample of custodially embattled mothers. Chesler found that "in court, 70 percent of the judges ordered children into paternal custody; 70 percent of the private arrangements also resulted in paternal custody. Within two years, 82 percent of all custody battles resulted in paternal custody" (p. 78).
12. Quoted in Judith Antonelli, "'No' to Surrogate Mothering," *Jewish Advocate*, January 22, 1987, 1.
13. Quoted in NOW compilation of positions articulated *In Re Baby M and Surrogate Arrangements*, NOW Legal Defense and Education Fund, 1987, 10, unpublished.
14. A. M. Rosenthal, "The Mother and the Judge," *New York Times*, April 5, 1987, E27.

15. C-SPAN videotape of the press conference on the founding of the National Coalition Against Surrogacy, *Surrogate Mothers,* August 31, 1987.

16. Brodribb, "ReproTech," 11.

17. Richard M. Titmuss, *The Gift Relationship: From Human Blood to Social Policy* (New York: Pantheon, 1971), 73.

18. Men donate sperm, of course, but sperm donation is simple and short-lived and procured from a pleasurable act, masturbation. Eggs are most often procured from an uncomfortable and unpleasant procedure, laparoscopy. As Andrea Dworkin has observed, comparing the donation of eggs and sperm—not to mention the woman's added "donation" of womb and body in surrogacy—is like comparing the giving of an eye to the shedding of a tear.

19. Titmuss designates this as the question that must be asked continually about gift relationships. See *Gift Relationship,* 221.

20. *Matter of Baby M.,* at 1227, 1264.

21. George J. Annas, "Death Without Dignity for Commercial Surrogacy: The Case of Baby M," *Hastings Center Report* 18, no. 2 (1988): 23, 21–24.

22. "Florida Woman to Be Surrogate Mother for Sister," *Greenfield Recorder,* November 12, 1985.

23. Stuart Rintoul and Jacke Allender, "Sister Surrogacy 'a Moral and Loving Act,'" *The Australian,* April 8, 1988, 1.

24. Linda Kirkman, "IVF, A Special Gift," *The Sun,* June 14, 1988, 8. See also the Kirkman sisters' book, *My Sister's Child: Maggie and Linda Kirkman, Their Own Story* (Victoria, Australia: Penguin Books, 1988), for a fuller discussion.

25. Eric Levin, "Motherly Love Works a Miracle," *People,* October 19, 1987, 43.

26. "S.D. Woman to Bear Daughter's Twins," *Providence Journal,* August 6, 1991, A1.

27. Sonia Humphrey, "Why Rent-a-Uterus Is a Noble Calling," *The Australian,* December 19, 1986.

28. Thomas and Barbara Bixton, "In Praise of Surrogacy," *Boston Globe,* April 24, 1987.

29. Louise Vandelac, "Mothergate: Surrogate Mothers, Linguistics, and Androcentric Engineering," originally published as "Mères porteuses ou mères deportées," trans. Jane Parniak and Lise Moisan, *Resources for Feminist Research/Documentation sur la recherche féministe* 15, no. 4 (1987): 47.

30. Nadine Brozan, "Egg Donation: Miraculous or Immoral?" *Providence Journal,* January 24, 1988, pp. B1, B8.

31. Renate Klein and Robyn Rowland, "Women as Test-Sites for Fertility Drugs," *Reproductive and Genetic Engineering* 1, no. 3 (1988): 251–73.

32. Leith appeared on the Ted Koppel "Nightline" show in January 1988. See also *Time* magazine, February 1, 1988, 49.

33. Barbara Katz Rothman, "On Donor Babies," *On the Issues*, Winter 1990, 39.

34. Katz Rothman, "On Donor Babies," 40.

35. Erwin Chargaff, "Engineering a Molecular Nightmare," *Nature* 327 (1987): 199–200.

36. Quoted in David Remnick, "Whose Life Is It, Anyway?" *Washington Post Magazine*, February 21, 1988, 41. The meaning here is that Angela Carder, even in knowing that she had cancer and would risk her health and life in conceiving, nevertheless elected to become pregnant.

37. Three years after Angela Carder died, a District of Columbia Court of Appeals wisely overturned the "hospital court's" decision. "The right of bodily integrity," said Judge John A. Perry, "is not extinguished simply because someone is ill, or even at death's door." The parents of Angela Carder received an out-of-court settlement, after suing the George Washington University Medical Center for malpractice and civil rights violations.

38. Caroline Whitbeck, "The Moral Implications of Regarding Women as People: New Perspectives on Pregnancy and Personhood," in *Abortion and the Status of the Fetus*, ed. William Bondeson et al. (Dordrecht: D. Reidel Publishing, 1983), 249.

39. "Ruling by Court Keeps Fetus Alive," *New York Times*, July 25, 1986.

40. Julien Murphy, "Postmortem Pregnancies: Legal and Ethical Issues in Sustaining Pregnancies in Brain-Dead Women" (Paper presented at the University of Connecticut National Women's Studies Association Meeting, June 1988), Storrs, Connecticut, 9–10, 13.

41. Quoted in Calvin Miller, "The Brain-Dead Could Be Surrogates, Say Scientists," *The Herald*, June 24, 1988, 1.

42. Jennifer Conley and Michael Pirrie, "Cain Willing to Change Law for IVF Baby," *The Age*, April 9, 1988.

43. Beverly Wildung Harrison, *Our Right to Choose: Toward a New Ethic of Abortion* (Boston: Beacon Press, 1983), 39–40.

44. Harrison, *Our Right to Choose*, 62.

45. Sarah Hoagland, *Lesbian Ethics: Toward New Value* (Palo Alto, CA: Institute of Lesbian Studies, 1988), 75.

46. Carol Gilligan, *In a Different Voice: Psychological Theory and Women's Development* (Cambridge: Harvard Univ. Press, 1982).

47. Catharine MacKinnon, *Feminism Unmodified: Discourses on Life and Law* (Cambridge: Harvard Univ. Press, 1987), 39.

48. Mary Daly, *Beyond God the Father: Toward a Philosophy of Women's Liberation* (Boston: Beacon Press, 1973), 100.

49. Lori B. Andrews, "Alternative Modes of Reproduction," in *Reproductive Laws for the 1990s: a Briefing Handbook*, ed. Nadine Taub and Sherrill Cohen (Newark: State Univ. Press, 1989), 269.

50. Emile Durkheim, *Suicide: A Study in Sociology*, trans. John A. Spaulding and George Simpson (New York: Free Press, 1951), 217–40.
51. Oral conversation with source who wishes to remain anonymous, June 1988.
52. Marie E. Meggitt, Letter to the Editor, "Surrogate Pain," *The Age*, June 5, 1986.
53. Marcel Mauss, *The Gift: Forms and Functions of Exchange in Archaic Societies*, trans. Ian Cunnison (New York: W. W. Norton, 1967), see especially chap. 1.
54. Testimony of Alejandra Muñoz, press conference on the founding of the National Coalition Against Surrogacy, Washington, DC, March 12, 1989.
55. Ronald Bailey, "Should I Be Allowed to Buy Your Kidney?" *Forbes*, May 28, 1990, 367.
56. Quoted in Robert Hanley, "Limits on Unpaid Surrogacy Backed," *New York Times*, March 12, 1989.
57. Hanley, "Limits on Unpaid Surrogacy Backed."
58. Quoted in Sally Heath, "Surrogacy to Be Outlawed as Health Ministers Unite," *The Age*, March 26, 1991.
59. Heath, "Surrogacy to Be Outlawed."
60. Australian Health Ministers Conference Secretariat, "No Legal Standing for Surrogacy" (Media release 1, joint meeting of the Australian Health Ministers Conference and the Council of Social Welfare Ministers, March 25, 1991).
61. Carol Mc Master (Final paper for Women's Studies 393, The New Reproductive and Genetic Technologies, University of Massachusetts, Spring 1989).
62. Quoted in "New Divorce Issue: Embryos' Status," *New York Times*, August 8, 1989, A11.
63. Quoted in "Preborn Children or Blastocysts?" *New York Times*, August 11, 1989, A26.
64. Quoted in "New Divorce Issue."
65. John Elson, "The Rights of Frozen Embryos," *Time*, July 1989, 63.
66. *York v. Jones*, 717 F. Supp. 421 (E.E.VA 1989).
67. This is my term to describe a political, legal, and medical context that increasingly focuses on the fetus as person, as patient, and on fetal rights. For further elaboration of this concept, see Janice G. Raymond, "Fetalists and Feminists: They Are Not the Same," in *Made to Order: The Myth of Reproductive and Genetic Progress*, ed. Patricia Spallone and Deborah Lynn Steinberg (New York: Pergamon, 1987), 58–66.
68. *Davis v. Davis*, 1990 Tenn. App. LEXIS 642 (13 September 1990), reported in Duncan Mansfield, "Embryo Ruling in Tennessee Is Overturned," *Boston Globe*, September 14, 1990, 3.

69. For a discussion of this decision, see Alexander Morgan Capron, "Parenthood and Frozen Embryos: More than Property and Privacy," *Hastings Center Report* 22, no. 5 (September–October 1992): 32–33.

70. John Stoltenberg, *Refusing to Be a Man: Essays on Sex and Justice* (Portland: Breitenbush Books, 1989), 96.

71. *In the Matter of the Unborn Child "H."* Vigo Circuit Ct. No. 84C01 8804 JP 185 (IN 1988).

72. Michael J. Weiss, "Equal Rights: Not for Women Only," *Glamour*, March 1989, 319.

73. Thomas Palmer, "Chantal vs. Jean-Guy: Canada's Abortion Case," *Boston Globe*, August 8, 1989, 5.

74. Palmer, "Canada's Abortion Case," 5.

75. James Barron, "Canada's Supreme Court Rejects Ex-Lover's Effort to Halt Abortion," *New York Times*, August 9, 1989, A8.

76. Sally Jacobs, "Man Breaks Silence in Embryo Case, Says He Opposes Single Parenthood," *Boston Globe*, August 11, 1989, 5.

77. "Surrogate's Lawsuit May Redefine Parenthood," *Washington Post*, August 15, 1990.

78. Quoted in Katha Pollitt, "When Is a Mother Not a Mother?" *Nation*, December 31, 1990, 842.

79. *Matter of Baby M.*, 525 A.2d 1169 (NJ Super. Ct. Ch. Div. 1987), rev'd, 537 A.2d 1227 (NJ 1988).

80. Catharine MacKinnon, "Reflections on Sex Equality Under Law," *Yale Law Journal* 100, no. 5 (March 1991): 1290, 1292.

81. Gena Corea, *The Mother Machine: Reproductive Technologies from Artificial Insemination to Artificial Wombs* (New York: Harper & Row, 1985), see especially chap. 11.

82. Pollitt, "When Is a Mother," 842.

83. "Study: Surrogate Moms Influence Genes of Fetus," *Durham Morning Herald*, November 22, 1990.

84. "Surrogate Moms."

85. "Excerpts from John Paul II's Apostolic Letter 'On the Dignity of Women,'" *New York Times*, October 1, 1988, 3.

86. The worldview that women exist for men and only in relation to them. See Janice G. Raymond, *A Passion for Friends: A Philosophy of Female Affection* (Boston: Beacon Press, 1986).

87. "Love Boat City on a New Course," *The Australian*, January 7, 1987.

88. "Around Asia," *International Herald Tribune*, May 5, 1988, 3. As we have seen in chapter 1, Singapore is not typical of non-Western countries. With the exception of Japan and Hong Kong, Singapore is the most Westernized and industrialized of the developing countries in Asia. In most developing countries, there is no maternal essentialism that flourishes in the service

of population proliferation. Rather, there are state-supported, Western-generated policies and practices of population control, and women are regarded as population polluters for having too many children.

89. Ben Wattenberg, *The Birth Dearth* (excerpt), *U.S. News & World Report*, June 22, 1987, 56–65.

90. "Too Late for Prince Charming?" *Newsweek*, June 2, 1986, 54–61. These figures, and the Harvard-Yale study itself, were later found to be contrived.

91. Since I wrote this, Susan Faludi's best-selling book, *Backlash*, has also debunked this study on similar and other grounds.

92. Jane Gross, "Single Women: Coping with a Void," *New York Times*, April 4, 1987.

93. Gross, "Single Women."

94. Blake's work, cited in Martha Gimenez, "Feminism, Pronatalism, and Motherhood," in *Mothering: Essays in Feminist Theory*, ed. Joyce Trebilcot (Totowa, NJ: Rowman and Allenheld, 1983), 288.

95. Gimenez, "Feminism, Pronatalism, and Motherhood," 291.

Chapter 3. A Critique of Reproductive Liberalism

1. These phrases can be found in many articles authored by Robertson. See, for example, John A. Robertson, "Procreative Liberty and the Control of Conception, Pregnancy, and Childbirth," *Virginia Law Review* 69, no. 3 (1983): 405–14.

2. *Matter of Baby M.*, 525 A.2d 1128, 1163–64 (NJ Super. Ct. Ch. Div. 1987), rev'd, 537 A.2d 1227 (NJ 1988).

3. *Matter of Baby M.*, at 1164.

4. *Matter of Baby M.*, at 1164.

5. Robertson, "Procreative Liberty," 405–14.

6. There are, obviously, a large number of fathers who do not fight for custody of their children, not wanting the responsibility and burden of raising children. Those who do fight for legal custody, in large measure, seek it because they set out to punish their exwives for, among other things, leaving them and/or for initiating divorce proceedings. See Phyllis Chesler, *Mothers on Trial: The Battle for Children and Custody* (New York: Harcourt Brace Jovanovich, 1991).

7. All statistics come from the United States listings, edited by Robin Morgan, *Sisterhood Is Global* (New York: Anchor Books, 1984), 696–705; this is a valuable sourcebook for statistics on women worldwide and includes an ample bibliography and documentation of other official sources for these statistics.

8. Lori B. Andrews, David Rankin, Nadine Taub, and Chris Flores, *General Dissent to the New Reproductive Technologies Advisory Committee to State Senator Connie Binsfield*, State of Michigan, March 1987, 1.

9. The Ethics Committee of the American Fertility Society, *Ethical Considerations of the New Reproductive Technologies, Fertility and Sterility*, Supplement 1, vol. 46, no. 3 (September 1986), especially 2S–7S. See p. iv for a listing of the members of the committee.

10. Kirsten Kozolanka, "Giving Up: The Choice That Isn't," in *Infertility: Women Speak Out About Their Experiences of Reproductive Medicine*, ed. Renate Klein (London: Pandora, 1989), 121, 128.

11. Beverly Wildung Harrison, *Our Right to Choose: Toward a New Ethic of Abortion* (Boston: Beacon Press, 1983), 9.

12. Sheila Jeffreys, *The Spinster and Her Enemies: Feminism and Sexuality 1880–1930* (London: Pandora, 1985), especially the introduction and chaps. 1 and 10.

13. Margaret Jackson, "The Political versus the Natural: Case Studies in the Struggle for Female Sexual Autonomy (1800–1940)" (Ph.D. diss., Univ. of Birmingham, England, 1990), especially chap. 7, "'Sex Freedom' or Female Sexual Autonomy?: Tensions and Divisions Within Feminism in the Late Nineteenth and Early Twentieth Centuries."

14. FINRRAGE is the acronym for the Feminist International Network of Resistance to Reproductive and Genetic Engineering. Originally called FINNRET, it was organized in Groningen, the Netherlands, in 1984 and now consists of over 1,000 members worldwide.

15. Nadine Taub and Sherrill Cohen, eds., *Reproductive Laws for the 1990s: A Briefing Handbook* (Newark: Women's Rights Litigation Clinic, Rutgers Law School, 1988); and Michelle Stanworth, ed., *Reproductive Technologies: Gender, Motherhood and Medicine* (Minneapolis: Univ. of Minnesota Press, 1988).

16. Michelle Stanworth, "The Deconstruction of Motherhood," in *Reproductive Technologies*, ed. Stanworth, 35.

17. Hilary Rose, "Victorian Values in the Test-Tube: The Politics of Reproductive Science and Technology," in *Reproductive Technologies*, ed. Stanworth, 152.

18. Shulamith Firestone, *The Dialectic of Sex: The Case for Feminist Revolution* (New York: William Morrow, 1970), esp. chap. 10.

19. Stanworth, "Deconstruction of Motherhood," 34.

20. Juliette Zipper and Selma Sevenhuijsen, "Surrogacy: Feminist Notions of Motherhood Reconsidered," in *Reproductive Technologies*, ed. Stanworth, 125.

21. Zipper and Sevenhuijsen, "Surrogacy," 126.

22. Alice Echols, "The New Feminism of Yin and Yang," in *Desire: The Politics of Sexuality*, ed. Ann Snitow et al. (London: Virago, 1984), 64, 66.

23. Lynne Segal, *Is the Future Female? Troubled Thoughts on Contemporary Feminism* (London: Virago, 1987), 3.

24. Liz Kelly, "The New Defeatism: A Review of *Is the Future Female?*" *Trouble and Strife* 11 (Summer 1987): 23–28.

25. See Patricia Spallone and Deborah Lynn Steinberg, *Made to Order: The Myth of Reproductive and Genetic Progress* (New York: Pergamon, 1987). The *Women's Review of Books* is a U.S. feminist publication whose coverage of both pornography and reproductive technologies has been almost totally authored by socialist liberals. Radical feminist work is unrelentingly assailed in the reviews and articles of this publication, which purports to be fair to all feminist viewpoints.

26. Rayna Rapp, "A Womb of One's Own: A Review of *Made to Order* and *Reproductive Technologies*," *The Women's Review of Books* 5, no. 7 (April 1988): 9–10.

27. Rebecca Albury, "'Babies on Ice': Aspects of Australian Press Coverage of IVF," *Australian Feminist Studies* 4 (Autumn 1987): 64.

28. Rapp, "Womb of One's Own," 9, uses this phrase to caricature the articles in *Made to Order*.

29. See Gena Corea and Cynthia De Wit, "Current Developments: German Police Raids," *Reproductive and Genetic Engineering* 1, no. 2 (1988): 191–94.

30. Rosalind Petchesky, "Fetal Images: The Power of Visual Culture in the Politics of Reproduction," *Feminist Studies* 13, no. 2 (1987): 280.

31. Rapp, "Womb of One's Own," 9.

32. Andrea Dworkin, *Right-Wing Women* (New York: Perigee, 1983), 94–95.

33. Ellen Carol Dubois and Linda Gordon, "Seeking Ecstasy on the Battlefield: Danger and Pleasure in Nineteenth Century Feminist Thought," in *Pleasure and Danger: Exploring Female Sexuality*, ed. Carol S. Vance (Boston: Routledge & Kegan Paul, 1984), 31–49.

34. Quoted in Sarah Snyder, "Baby M Trial Hears Closing Arguments," *Boston Globe*, March 13, 1987.

35. Lori Andrews, "Alternative Modes of Reproduction," in *Reproductive Laws for the 1990s: A Briefing Handbook* (Newark: Women's Rights Litigation Clinic, Rutgers Law School, 1988), 293.

36. Michelle Stanworth, "The Deconstruction of Motherhood," in *Reproductive Technologies: Gender, Motherhood, and Medicine*, ed. Michelle Stanworth (Oxford: Polity Press, 1987; Minneapolis: Univ. of Minnesota Press, 1988), 17.

37. *Matter of Baby M.*, 537 A.2d 1227, 1250 (NJ 1988).

38. FACT (Feminist Anti-Censorship Taskforce et al.), Brief Amici Curiae, No. 84-3147, in the U.S. Court of Appeals, 7th Circuit (Southern District of Indiana, 1985), at 4, brackets mine.

39. See Ellen Willis, "Feminism, Moralism, and Pornography," in *Desire: The Politics of Sexuality*, ed. Ann Snitow et al. (London: Virago, 1983), especially 84. Willis writes, "A woman who enjoys pornography (even if that means enjoying a rape fantasy) is in a sense a rebel, insisting on an aspect of her sexuality that has been defined as a male preserve. Insofar as pornography glorifies male supremacy and sexual alienation, it is deeply reactionary. But

in rejecting sexual repression and hypocrisy—which have inflicted even more damage on women than on men—it expresses a radical impulse." Willis tries to have it both ways. In effect she is saying to women, use it and be abused by it. But the two cannot be separated; there is not one kind of pornography that frees women and another that harms us.

40. Andrea Dworkin and Catharine A. MacKinnon, *Pornography and Civil Rights: A New Day for Women's Equality* (Minneapolis: Organizing Against Pornography, 1988), 43.

41. Katharina Stens, "Give Me Children, Or Else I Die," in *Infertility*, ed. Klein, 11.

42. Kathleen Barry, "The New Historical Syntheses: Women's Biography," *Journal of Women's History* 1, no. 3 (Winter 1990): 80, 84, 87.

Chapter 4. The Marketing of the New Reproductive Technologies: Medicine, the Media, and the Idea of Progress

1. Dorothy Nelkin, *Selling Science: How the Press Covers Science and Technology* (New York: W. H. Freeman, 1987), 173–74.

2. Edward S. Herman and Noam Chomsky, *Manufacturing Consent: The Political Economy of the Mass Media* (New York: Pantheon, 1988), 23.

3. Nelkin, *Selling Science*, 173–74.

4. Keith Schneider, "Repro Madness," *New Age Journal*, January 1986, 34, 36.

5. Schneider, "Repro Madness," 36.

6. Susan Downie, "Enlightened Beginnings: Advanced Embryology May Result in Healthier Babies," *Vogue Australia*, January 1988, 20.

7. Quoted in Dan McDonnell, "IVF Professor Blasts Critics," *The Sun*, June 8, 1988. Encoded in this statement, but not articulated by Wood, is that these conceptions only succeed to the small extent that they do because women subject themselves to more pain, more intervention, more risk, and more bodily intrusion.

8. Michael Beach and Jane Howard, "IVF Babies Four Times More Likely to Die at Birth," *The Australian*, November 20, 1985.

9. Herman and Chomsky, *Manufacturing Consent*, 38–42.

10. "Your A-Z Guide to Health," *U.S. News & World Report*, June 18, 1990, 90.

11. Debra Sorrentino Larson, "Surrogate Mother Extols 'Joy of Life' in Novel Experience," *Los Angeles Times*, January 1, 1987.

12. Mark Schwed, "Surrogate Mothers of Invention," *Los Angeles Herald Examiner*, May 23, 1988.

13. *National Women's Health Network News*, March 1992, 2.

14. *National Women's Health Network News*, March 1992, 3.

15. Dunstan McNichol, "Citing Risk to Safety, FDA Bans Most Silicone Breast Implants," *Boston Globe*, April 17, 1992, 3.

16. Formal Comment of the American Society of Plastic and Reconstructive Surgeons filed with the FDA on July 1, 1982, and quoted in Felicity Barringer, "Many Surgeons Reassure Their Patients on Implants," *New York Times*, January 29, 1992, C12, emphasis mine.

17. Philip J. Hilts, "Maker of Implants Balked at Tests, Its Records Show," *New York Times*, January 13, 1992, B10.

18. Judy Foreman, "Women and Silicone: A History of Risk," *Boston Sunday Globe*, January 19, 1992, 1.

19. Loretta J. Ross, "The Shot Felt Around the World," *Vital Signs: News from the National Black Women's Health Project*, Winter 1990, 11.

20. "Indian Agency on Contraception," *New York Times*, August 7, 1987.

21. A 1989 study done by the Public Citizen Health Research Group, part of Ralph Nader's organization, documented this finding using overall cesarian rates from forty-one states and individual hospital rates for cesarians in thirty states, the first time this has been done. "These avoidable operations cost about $1 billion a year and result in 25,000 serious postsurgical infections that require an extra 1.1 million days in the hospital. . . ." See Richard A. Knox, "Half of Caesarean Births Are Needless, Group Says," *Boston Globe*, January 27, 1989, p. 4. One month earlier, a study by two doctors published in the *New England Journal of Medicine* indicated that the U.S. cesarian rate could be cut in half without harm to babies. This study admitted that "the most important nonmedical reason for increasing Caesarean rates is convenience [to doctors]." See Richard Knox, "Study Indicates US Caesarean Rate Can be Halved Without Harm to Babies," *Boston Globe*, December 8, 1988, 22.

22. See Betsy Lehman, "Doubts Growing Over Fetal Monitors," *Boston Globe*, October 8, 1990, 59, 61. Lehman cites an editorial in the *New England Journal of Medicine* calling fetal monitoring "a disappointing story." This editorial in turn cited half a dozen studies involving a total of 17,510 infants, not one study finding that electronic monitoring did a better job of saving babies or improving health than frequent checks with a stethoscope. Too often the monitors indicate problems where none exist and, therefore, increase the number of unnecessary cesarian deliveries.

23. U.S. Public Health Service, Department of Health and Human Services, "Caring for a Future: The Content of Prenatal Care" (September 1989). Their phone number is: 301/443-4100.

24. Quoted in Nelkin, *Selling Science*, 45. This discussion of the early history and press coverage of ERT draws heavily on Nelkin's work.

25. Robert A. Wilson, *Feminine Forever* (New York: M. Evans, 1966).

26. His promotional work was featured in a 1969 issue of the *Ladies' Home Journal* and in his own book, *The Pill: Fact and Fallacies* (New York: Delacorte Press, 1969).

27. Nelkin, *Selling Science*, 47.

28. Nelkin cites women's magazines, such as *Vogue* in 1974, that continued such promotional coverage, *Selling Science*, 47.

29. Two critical studies appearing in the NEJM were: Donald C. Smith et al., "Association of Exogenous Estrogen and Endometrial Carcinoma," *The New England Journal of Medicine* 293, no. 23 (December 4, 1975): 1164–67; and Harry K. Ziel and William D. Finkle, "Increased Risk of Endometrial Carcinoma Among Users of Conjugated Estrogens," 293, no. 23 (December 4, 1975): 1167–70. The day after these studies were published, the *New York Times* reported on the attitudes of gynecologists who, after learning about the estrogen risks, nonetheless stated they would prescribe it as usual.

30. Nelkin, *Selling Science*, 47.

31. Anne Rochon Ford, "Hormones: Getting Out of Hand," in *Adverse Effects: Women and the Pharmaceutical Industry*, ed. Kathleen McDonnell (Penang, Malaysia: International Organization of Consumers Unions Regional Office for Asia and the Pacific, 1986), 33.

32. Michael Specter, "Hormone Use in Menopause Tied to Cancer," *Washington Post*, August 3, 1989, A1.

33. Gina Kolata, in the *New York Times*, September 12, 1991, B11; Jerry E. Bishop, "Doubt Remains About Estrogen for Menopause," *Wall Street Journal*, September 12, 1991, B1.

34. Mike Rayner, "Experiments on Embryos: Stick to the Facts," *New Scientist*, February 27, 1986, 54.

35. Diana Dutton, *Worse than the Disease: Pitfalls of Medical Progress* (Cambridge: Cambridge Univ. Press, 1988), 4.

36. See, for example, A. Cochrane, *Effectiveness and Efficiency: Random Reflections on Health Services* (London: Nuffield Provincial Hospitals Trust, 1971); and Stanley Joel Reiser, *Medicine and the Reign of Technology* (Cambridge: Cambridge Univ. Press, 1978).

37. Rene Dubos, *Mirage of Health: Utopias, Progress, and Biological Change* (New York: Harper & Row, Perennial Library, 1959), 22–23.

38. Thomas McKeown, *The Role of Medicine: Dream, Mirage, or Nemesis?* (Princeton: Princeton Univ. Press, 1979).

39. Dutton, *Worse than the Disease*, 25.

40. David Baltimore, "Keynote Address" (AAAS Annual Meeting, Boston, Massachusetts, February 11, 1988, Press Release).

41. Baltimore, "Keynote Address," 2.

42. Michael Pirrie, "Embryo Controls Block Medical Advances, Says Academic," *Age*, August 8, 1986.

43. Quoted by Keith Schneider, "Repro Madness," 72.

44. Marsden Wagner, Director of Maternal and Child Health, European Regional Office of the World Health Organization (WHO), in an address to the Sixth World Congress on In Vitro Fertilization and Alternate Assisted

Reproduction in Jerusalem, Israel, April 3, 1989. Excerpted by Gena Corea, "Current Developments and Issues: A Summary," *Reproductive and Genetic Engineering* 2, no. 3 (1989): 253–54. Although Wagner's work is often cited as *the* recognized critical expert in the media on technological reproduction, he relies on critical feminist sources cited throughout this book, sources who have not received the acknowledgment that Wagner, as a reputable doctor and official of the WHO, receives.

45. Wagner, in Corea, "Current Developments," 253–54.
46. WHO Summary Report, "Consultation on the Place of *in vitro* Fertilization in Infertility Care" (World Health Organization Regional Office for Europe, Copenhagen, June 18–22, 1990), 1–7.
47. WHO Summary Report (1990), 2–3.
48. Herman and Chomsky, *Manufacturing Consent*, 18.
49. Herman and Chomsky, *Manufacturing Consent*, 22.
50. Robert S. Cowen, "Garbage Under Glass: What Are Scientists Dishing Out?" *Technology Review* 81 (November 1979): 10–11.
51. Ethics Committee of the American Fertility Society, "Ethical Considerations of the New Reproductive Technologies," *Fertility and Sterility* 46, no. 3, Supplement 1 (September 1986): 78.
52. Ethics Committee, "Ethical Considerations," 56S.
53. Gena Corea, "Who May Have Children and Who May Not," in *Reconstructing Babylon*, ed. H. Patricia Hynes (Bloomington: Indiana Univ. Press, 1991), 71.
54. Steven Findlay, "The Surrogate Mother: Do We Need Standards?" *USA Today*, September 6, 1986, D1.
55. Langdon Winner, *Autonomous Technology: Technics-out-of-Control as a Theme in Political Thought* (Cambridge: MIT Press, 1977), 25.
56. Jacques Ellul, *The Technological Society*, trans. John Wilkinson (New York: Alfred A. Knopf, 1964), 85.
57. Dutton, *Worse than the Disease*, 206.
58. Cited in Dutton, *Worse than the Disease*, 215.
59. Richard Kay, "Three Babies 'Sacrificed' for Sake of Twins," *Daily Mail*, June 21, 1986, emphasis mine.
60. Christine Overall, "Selective Termination of Pregnancy and Women's Reproductive Autonomy," *Hastings Center Report*, May/June 1990, 8.
61. Overall, "Selective Termination of Pregnancy," 8.
62. Dan Chu, "A Dramatic Medical Rescue Saves the Schellin Twins from Their Mother's Nightmare Pregnancy," *People*, May 9, 1988, 51.
63. Chu, "Dramatic Medical Rescue," 53, 55.
64. H. Patricia Hynes, "Reconstructing Babylon: Women and Appropriate Technology" (Keynote address given at Nordic Conference on Women, Environment and Development, Norwegian Research Council for Science

and the Humanities, the Secretariat for Women and Research, University of Oslo, Center for Research on Women, Oslo, Norway, November 1990), 20.

65. Daniel Callahan, *What Kind of Life? The Limits of Medical Progress* (New York: Simon & Schuster, 1989).
66. U.S. Congress, H.R. 1161, 102d Cong., 1st sess., 1–182.
67. H.R. 1161, Subtitle F, Federal Employee Family Building Act, sec. 252, at 11–13.
68. H.R. 1161, Subtitle F, Contraceptive and Infertility Research Centers Act, sec. 151, at 7–10.
69. "Calls IVF Safe but Questions Efficacy Rates," *Ob. Gyn. News*, September 1, 1987, 3.

Chapter 5. The International Traffic in Women, Children, and Fetuses

1. Louise Vandelac, "Mothergate: Surrogate Mothers, Linguistics, and Androcentric Engineering," trans. Jane Parniak and Lise Moisan, *Resources for Feminist Research/Documentation sur la recherche féministe* 15, no. 4 (1987): 259.
2. Kathleen Barry was the first to document extensively the prostitution networks and sexual trafficking in women globally and to make connections between various forms of what she has called "female sexual slavery." See Kathleen Barry, *Female Sexual Slavery* (Englewood Cliffs, NJ: Prentice-Hall, 1979; paperback reprint, New York: New York Univ. Press, 1984).
3. Quoted in Mike Breen, "Olympics Fuel a Dream More Potent than Fear of Aids," *The Guardian*, July 26, 1988.
4. See Kathleen Barry et al., *International Feminism: Networking Against Female Sexual Slavery*, Report of the Global Feminist Workshop to Organize Against Traffic in Women, Rotterdam, the Netherlands, April 6–15, 1983 (New York: International Women's Tribune Centre, 1984), for documentation of the extensive links between the prostitution, sex tourism, and mail order bride industry.
5. Bill Mellor, "Evil 'Baby Farms' Exposed," *Sunday Herald*, April 13, 1986.
6. Anti-Slavery Society for the Protection of Human Rights, "Sale of Children" (Report to the United Nations Working Group on Slavery, 1982), 1.
7. Mellor, "Evil 'Baby Farms' Exposed."
8. Dexter Cruez, "Baby Trade Booming in Sri Lanka," *Sydney Morning Herald*, January 30, 1987.
9. Cruez, "Baby Trade Booming."
10. "Women — Guatemala," *Latinamerican Press*, July 20, 1989, 6.
11. Roberta Walker, "The Market in Babies," *Canadian Lawyer*, February 1987, 22.

12. One lawyer advertises in *Philadelphia Magazine* that he will provide international infant adoptions free of the regulatory hassle of U.S. court appearances. He also offers no waiting list, an original birth certificate to be issued in the adoptive parents' name, and the necessary federal and state approvals. See classifieds, "International Infant Adoptions by Private Attorney," *Philadelphia Magazine,* September 1990.

13. Walker, "The Market in Babies," 22.

14. Widespread advertising by lawyers offering private international adoptions is commonplace in U.S. publications. Advertising is also used by couples to solicit babies in the United States. Many state laws forbid lawyers to directly find babies for clients so, instead, lawyers coach couples on how to place the ads, set up special phone lines in their homes to field inquiries from pregnant women or others, and then refer the more suitable callers to the lawyers who do the rest of the work. Couples pay to attend seminars where they can pick up tips on how to go about advertising. Advice is usually to "concentrate on small, rural area papers rather than those in big cities. 'You're looking for a population group where they may not be as sophisticated in terms of information about birth control, a strong fundamentalist area where the anti-abortion message would be quite strong and there might be a stigma against single mothers,'" according to Bob Secter, "Looking for Baby in the Want Ads," *San Francisco Chronicle,* June 9, 1987. Campus newspapers are also targeted, since the presumption is that young college women who become pregnant are likely not to raise the children.

   On the national front, the Child Welfare League estimates that one-third of the annual 50,000 private adoptions in the United States that do not involve relatives take place outside traditional adoption agencies. "Texas leads all states in the number of adoptions: more than 8,100 in 1986, 75 percent of which were private," says Howard La Franchi, "Couples Target Texas in Search of Newborns," *Christian Science Monitor* 81, no. 94 (April 11, 1989): 12.

15. La Franchi, "Couples Target Texas," 13.

16. For excerpts from the Joint Women's Programme study, see Asha Rames and Philomena H. P., "The Devadasi Problem," in Barry et al., *International Feminism,* 82–87. The Joint Women's Programme has campaigned successfully in India to tighten the penalties for procuring women and has done extensive research with women in various types of prostitution, publishing work that exposes the deeply embedded cultural practices perpetuating prostitution in India.

17. "Women Sold Like Cheese Says Study," *Khaleej Times,* October 21, 1986, 9.

18. Redd Barna (Norwegian Save the Children Organization), "The Sexual Exploitation of Children in Developing Countries" (Preliminary Summary, Oslo, June, 1989), 8.

19. Piet Stoffelen, Rapporteur, *Parliamentary Assembly Report on the Traffic in Children and Other Forms of Child Exploitation*, Council of Europe, September 10, 1987, 3, 8. His report is based on the findings of Interpol, the Anti-Slavery Society, the International Labour Organisation, various UN groups, adoption agencies, and local newspaper reports. It is also important to note that Stoffelen's report reiterates what the Coalition Against Trafficking in Women had documented earlier (1983–84) in its own report on networking against female sexual slavery. See Barry et al., *International Feminism*.

20. Stoffelen, *Traffic in Children*, 7. Kathleen Barry also writes, "When child prostitution is separated from that of exploitation of adult women . . . the invisibility surrounding the violation of women serves to perpetuate the exploitation of children." As a result of different standards used to differentiate the exploitation of children from that of adult women, one country after another is trying to define children as adults, thus making more and more children available to sexual exploitation by lowering the age of consent and assisting pimps and procurers. "There are special considerations we must make when we face child prostitution and pornography. The physical and psychological effects of sexual exploitation . . . on the young may well be more severe than the effects of such practices on adult women. Nevertheless, an act which is intended to degrade, humiliate and exploit is a violation of the *human being*, whatever her age, culture, race or condition." See Kathleen Barry, "The Opening Paper: International Politics of Female Sexual Slavery," in Kathleen Barry et al., *International Feminism*, 30.

21. "Venta mundial de niños argentinos," *La Razon*, October 6, 1986, 19. I thank Rita Arditti for drawing my attention to this article (in English, "World Sale of Argentinian Children") and for providing the translation of relevant passages.

22. See Gena Corea and Cynthia De Wit, "Current Developments and Issues," *Reproductive and Genetic Engineering* 1, no. 2 (1988): 191; also Steven Dickman, "West German Protest over US Surrogacy Company," *Nature* 329 (1987): 577.

23. Gena Corea, *The Mother Machine: Reproductive Technologies from Artificial Insemination to Artificial Wombs* (New York: Harper & Row, 1985), 214.

24. Francisco J. Pilotti, "Intercountry Adoption: A View from Latin America," *Child Welfare* 64, no. 1 (January–February 1985): 27.

25. Randall Richard, "Reporter, Photographer Track Americans in Search of Children," *Providence Journal*, May 3, 1987, A18.

26. Pilotti, "Intercountry Adoption," 29–30.

27. Centre for the Protection of Children's Rights, quoted in *Asiaweek*, February 5, 1988, 14.

28. Peter Spinks, "Bangkok's Baby Snatchers," in "Children for Sale," *South*, December 1987, 10.

8

29. Anti-Slavery Society, "Sale of Children," 2.
30. One need not only look to Third World countries for these results of milita-
    rism. After World War II, large numbers of German children were adopted
    in other countries, particularly in the United States. Many were orphans
    whose parents had died as a result of the war; many were the children of
    mothers who lacked the strength and resources after the war to raise them;
    and many were the children of women made pregnant by occupying sol-
    diers. Of the latter group, many were interracial children, who did not fit
    into the "post-Aryan" German society. See the report by the International
    Social Service, German Branch, "Problems Concerning the Adoption from
    Countries of the 'Third World'" (Frankfurt am Main, May 17–19, 1982), 4.
31. Jean-Marie Simon, *Guatemala: Eternal Spring, Eternal Tyranny* (New York:
    W. W. Norton, 1987), 173.
32. Quoted in *Enfoprensa USA*, January 16, 1989, 2.
33. Isabel Santa Maria, "Trafficking in Children: A Horrendous Crime," *Barri-
    cada*, April 21, 1987, 2.
34. Stoffelen, *Traffic in Children*, 2–3; see also Spinks, "Bangkok's Baby
    Snatchers," 9.
35. Marlise Simons, "Abductions in Salvador Fill a Demand: Adoption," *New
    York Times*, December 17, 1985.
36. Alain Feder and Antoine Garapon, "Enquête sur un éventuel trafic d'or-
    ganes d'enfants," quoted in the *International Children's Rights Monitor* 5,
    no. 4 (1988): 2.
37. Simons, "Abductions in Salvador"; see also "International Charges of Child
    Trafficking," *Central America Report*, November 18, 1988, 359; see also
    Stoffelen, *Traffic in Children*, 2–3.
38. Feder and Garapon, "Trafic d'organes d'enfants," 2.
39. Feder and Garapon, "Trafic d'organes d'enfants," 2.
40. NGO Forum: *NGO/UNICEF Newsletter*, December 1984, 1.
41. Roxanna Pastor, "The Honduran Baby Market," *Sojourner: The Women's
    Forum*, May 1989, 19.
42. "Adoption from Abroad," *Newsweek*, June 1988, 44.
43. Angela Romito, "Stopping the Traffic of Children by Regulating Adoption,"
    O Globo, September 7, 1986.
44. Stoffelen, *Traffic in Children*, 5.
45. Gena Corea, unpublished interview with John Stehura, December 1987.
46. Corea, unpublished interview with Stehura.
47. William Robinson and Kent Norsworthy, *David and Goliath: The U.S. War
    Against Nicaragua* (New York: Monthly Review Press, 1987), 134.
48. Stoffelen, *Traffic in Children*, 5.
49. Frank Walker, "Worldwide Child Trade Fuelled by Big Money," *Sun Herald*,
    June 29, 1986.

50. Walker, "Worldwide Child Trade."
51. Walker, "Worldwide Child Trade."
52. Ahilemeh Jonet, "Trafficking in Children for Intercountry Adoptions: Causes and Rationality" (Unpublished paper prepared for the Fourth Biennial Congress on the Fate and Hope of the Earth, Managua, Nicaragua, June 5–9, 1989), 1.
53. Mi Ok Bruining, "Challenging the Lies of International Adoption by White Lesbians and Gays," *Color Life,* 1 (1992), 22–23.
54. Maria Josefina Becker, "The Pressure to Abandon," *International Children's Rights Monitor,* May 1988, 12–13, emphasis mine.
55. Jonet, "Trafficking in Children," 6–14.
56. Jonet, "Trafficking in Children," 17.
57. Jonet, "Trafficking in Children," 35–36.
58. Jonet, "Trafficking in Children," 32.
59. George and Laurel Harper, "For the Love of a Child," *Cincinnati Enquirer,* May 6, 1984, A12–A16.
60. Becker, "Pressure to Abandon," 12.
61. Danilo D. Antunez, "Niños hondureños despedazados para traficar con sus organos," *La Tribuna,* January 2, 1987; see also translation in *International News,* January 6, 1987, 1.
62. Michel Raffoul, "Chair humaine à vendre," *Jeune Afrique,* May 11, 1988, 50–54, translation mine.
63. "¿Ocurrió en el pasado?" *Tiempo,* January 9, 1987, emphasis mine.
64. "Rescatarón a catorce niños," *Prensa Libre,* February 5, 1987, 55.
65. "Otros 16 niños rescatados," *Prensa Libre,* March 4, 1987, 39.
66. "International Charges of Trafficking," *Central America Report* 18 (1988): 358–65.
67. Santa Maria, "Trafficking in Children," 2.
68. "Adoptions for Organ Transplants: In Search of the Truth," *International Children's Rights Monitor,* April 1, 1987, 16.
69. "DCI and the Allegations of Trafficking in Organs," *International Children's Rights Monitor,* April 3, 1987, 4–5.
70. "Allegations of Trafficking," 5.
71. "A luz exportación de niños para 'destace,'" *El Gráfico,* January 24, 1988.
72. "Israel respetuoso de la vida," *El Gráfico,* January 27, 1988.
73. Guatemalan Health Rights Support Project Communique, "Resolution to Urgent Action of 2/23/88," April 22, 1988.
74. "Madre y Rosita Huyen por miedo a mafia," *El Comerrio,* November 14, 1988, 2–3.
75. John Goshko, "Nailing Disinformation: The Slum-Child Tale," *Washington Post,* August 26, 1988, A19.
76. Goshko, "Nailing Disinformation," A19.

77. Janice G. Raymond, telephone interview with John Goshko, *Washington Post* reporter, May 10, 1989.

78. Goshko, "Nailing Disinformation," A19.

79. Luis Mauro of Reuters in Asunción, "Babies Kidnapped for US Organ Banks," *The Daily Telegraph,* August 9, 1988.

80. Goshko, "Nailing Disinformation," A20.

81. "U.S. Says Moscow Spread Lies about Baby-Organ Trafficking," *Washington Post,* October 21, 1988, 28.

82. Santa Maria, "Trafficking in Children," 1987.

83. "Brazilian Children Sold for Transplants," *Guardian,* September 30, 1990, 10; also Franco Scottoni, "Bambini ridotti a pezzi di ricambio," trans. as "Children Reduced to Spare Parts," *la Repubblica,* September 17, 1990, 19. I thank Silvia Federici of Hofstra University for her translation of this Italian article into English.

84. "Brazilian Children Sold," 10.

85. "Latin Bishops: No to Child Killing," *The Dialog,* May 31, 1991, 2.

86. "Latin Bishops," 2.

87. Vivek Chaudhary, "Argentina Uncovers Patients Killed for Organs," *British Medical Journal* 304 (April 25, 1992): 1073–74.

88. Mariano N. Castex, "Argentina: Alleged Murders at Psychiatric Institute," *The Lancet* 339, (May 2, 1992): 1102.

89. Castex, "Argentina: Alleged Murders," 1102.

90. The term *middle knowledge* was used by Robert Jay Lifton to explain the kind of belief and disbelief that people had about the Nazi genocide. "There seems to be something murderous in the air, stories of mass killing that are both disbelieved and believed." See *The Nazi Doctors* (New York: Basic Books, 1986), 489.

91. Nancy Scheper-Hughes, "Bodies, Death, and the State: Violence and the Taken-for-Granted World" (Paper presented at a symposium of the American Ethnological Society, Atlanta, Georgia, April 28, 1990), 13.

92. Louise Palmer, "'Baby Parts' Myth Explained," *New Directions for Women,* March/April 1991, 8.

93. Helmut L. Karcher, "No More Living Donors in Munich," *British Medical Journal* 297 (1988): 1292.

94. Noam Chomsky, "Victors I," *Z Magazine* 3, no. 11 (November 1990): 15; "Victors II," *Z Magazine* 4, no. 1 (January 1991): 10.

95. Regula Bott, "Organhandel, Personlichkeitsrechte, Kinderhandel und kriminelle Organentnahme insbesondere bei Kindern in der dritten Welt," *Mitglied de Deutschen Bundestages,* December 20, 1988, 1–8. I thank Renate Klein for assisting me with the translation of this document from German to English.

96. Ronald Bailey, "Should I Be Allowed to Buy Your Kidney?" *Forbes,* May 28, 1990, 370.

97. Quoted in Margaret Rice, Editor's Column, *Medical Observer,* January 22, 1993.

98. Bailey, "Buy Your Kidney," 367.

99. Karcher, "No More Living Donors in Munich," 1292.

100. Quoted in Raffoul, "Chair humaine à vendre," 50, translation mine.

101. Raffoul, "Chair humaine à vendre," 50.

102. Raffoul, "Chair humaine à vendre," 50, 51.

103. Roland Girard, *Le Fruit de vos entrailles* (Paris: Editions Suger, 1985).

104. Girard, *Le Fruit de vos entrailles.*

105. "Embryos to Lipstick?" *New Scientist,* October 10, 1985, 21.

106. "Foetuses Sold to Labs, BBC Says," *Sydney Morning Herald,* November 1, 1985.

107. Peter McCullagh, *The Foetus as Transplant Donor: Scientific, Social, and Ethical Perspectives* (New York: John Wiley & Sons, 1988).

108. Transcript of ABC News, "Nightline," January 6, 1988, show no. 1728, 4.

109. R. Weiss, "Fetal-Cell Transplants Show Few Benefits," *Science News* 134 (November 5, 1988): 324.

110. Georgina Ferry, "New Cells for Old Brains," *New Scientist,* March 24, 1988, 58.

111. Georgina Ferry, "Swedes Voice Pessimism About Fetal Transplants," *New Scientist,* June 16, 1988, 34.

112. Weiss, "Fetal-Cell Transplants," 324.

113. Quoted in Weiss, "Fetal-Cell Transplants," 324.

114. Roger Lewin, "Caution Continues over Transplants," *Science,* December 9, 1988, 1379.

115. Beverly Merz, "Neurologists Join Neurosurgeons in Urging Restraint in Parkinson's Surgery," *Journal of the American Medical Association* 261, no. 20 (May 26, 1989): 2929.

116. Ferry, "New Cells for Old Brains," 88.

117. Eugene B. Brody, "Human Rights Aspects of Transactions in Body Parts and Human Fetuses" (Prepared for UNESCO, Division of Human Rights and Peace, Paris, France, April 1990), 15, 8.

118. Gina Kolata, "More U.S. Curbs Urged in the Use of Fetal Tissue," *New York Times,* November 19, 1991, 38.

119. Kolata, "More U.S. Curbs Urged," 38.

120. Stuart Newman, quoted in Rick Weiss, "Forbidding Fruits of Fetal-Cell Research," *Science News* 134 (November 5, 1988): 297.

121. Alan Fine, "The Ethics of Fetal Tissue Transplants," *Hastings Center Report* (June/July 1988), 6. Although the author supports fetal tissue transplants and research, the figures he provides in this article raise serious questions about the limits of the supply of fetal tissue. See also McCullagh, *The Foetus as Transplant Donor.*

122. Kolata, "More U.S. Curbs Urged," 38.

123. Susanna Rodell, "The Brain Cell Dilemma," *The Herald*, May 5, 1988.

124. "U.S. Panel Affirms Stand on Research on Tissue of Fetuses," *New York Times*, December 7, 1988, B13.

125. Andrew Veitch, "Doctors Fear World Trade in Stockpiled Embryos," *Guardian*, October 5, 1987, 4.

126. Calvin Miller, "IVF 'Out of Control' as European Embryo Stockpiles Grow," *The Herald*, January 23, 1990.

127. I stress the role of feminists in this realm because, for the most part, feminists have not articulated the role of the fetus in relation to the pregnant woman other than to deny its personhood and rights vis-à-vis the woman. It is necessary at the same time, however, to spell out the political relation of woman and fetus, and feminists should take the lead in defining this relationship. For a further development of this political relation, see Catharine MacKinnon, "Reflections on Sex Equality Under Law," *The Yale Law Journal* 100, no. 5 (March 1991): 1281–1328.

128. MacKinnon, "Sex Equality Under Law," 1316. MacKinnon cites Adrienne Rich's formulation of this relationship from *Of Woman Born:* "The child I carry for nine months can be defined *neither* as me nor as not-me." MacKinnon then credits Lynn Smith with suggesting that Rich's definition be stated in the affirmative.

129. *Commonweal*, December 1988, 676.

130. Emanuel Thorne, "Trade in Human Tissue Needs Regulation," *Wall Street Journal*, August 19, 1987.

131. "The Flesh Peddlers," *The Progressive*, October 1987, 10.

132. Quoted in Rick Weiss, "Bypassing the Ban," *Science News* 136 (December 9, 1989): 378.

133. Testimony of Janice G. Raymond, NIH *Reauthorization*, Hearings before the Subcommittee on Health and the Environment, 102d Congress, 1st sess. April 15, 1991, "Fetal Tissue Transplantation Research" (H.R. 1532), Serial No. 102–24; see also Philip J. Hilts, "Fetal Tissue Use: Personal Agony in Medical First," *New York Times*, April 16, 1991.

134. Brody, "Human Rights Aspects of Transactions in Body Parts and Human Fetuses," 40.

Chapter 6. International Human Rights, Integrity, and Legal Frameworks

1. Maria Mies, "From the Individual to the Dividual: In the Supermarket of 'Reproductive Alternatives,'" *Reproductive and Genetic Engineering* 1, no. 3 (1988): 236.

2. Mies, "From the Individual," 236.

3. Deborah Cameron and Liz Fraser, "The Liberal Organ: Porn in *The Guardian*," *Trouble and Strife* 4 (Winter 1984): 26.

4. Sherene Razack, "Wrong Rights: Feminism Applied to Law," *Le Bulletin/ Newsletter,* Institut Simone de Beauvoir, 10, no. 1 (1990): 13.

5. Mies, "From the Individual," 225–37.

6. Maria Mies, "Self-Determination: The End of a Utopia?" Resources for Feminist Research/Documentation sur la recherche feministe 18, no. 3 (September 1989): 52.

7. Michael Ignatieff, *The Needs of Strangers* (London: Chatto and Windus, 1984), 38.

8. Patricia Williams, *The Alchemy of Race and Rights: Diary of a Law Professor* (Cambridge: Harvard Univ. Press, 1991), 153; emphasis mine.

9. Williams, *Alchemy of Race and Rights,* 153, 154.

10. Williams, *Alchemy of Race and Rights,* 164.

11. Testimony of John A. Robertson in *Human Embryo Transfer,* Hearings before the Subcommittee of Investigations and Oversight of the Committee on Science and Technology, 98th Cong., 2d sess., August 8–9, 1984, doc. 142.

12. Kathleen Barry was the first to point this out. Her remarks on women's dignity and integrity underlying human rights claims have been incorporated into the final report of the International Meeting of Experts on the Social and Cultural Causes of Prostitution and Strategies for the Struggle Against Procuring and Sexual Exploitation of Women, UNESCO, Division of Human Rights and Peace, Madrid, Spain, March 1986, 1–18.

13. Warren Lee Holleman, *The Human Rights Movement: Western Values and Theological Perspectives* (New York: Praeger, 1987), 27.

14. George H. Brand, quoted in Holleman, *Human Rights Movement,* 98.

15. See, for example, the first Amnesty International feature story dedicated to women, entitled "Women in the Front Line for Human Rights," *Amnesty Action,* March/April 1991, 1, 3.

16. Much of what happens to women, such as being prostituted or used for breeding, also happens as a result of national and political conflicts.

17. Catharine MacKinnon, *Feminism Unmodified: Discourses on Life and Law* (Cambridge: Harvard Univ. Press, 1987), 40–41.

18. See MacKinnon's essay, "Not a Moral Issue," in *Feminism Unmodified,* 146–62.

19. MacKinnon, *Feminism Unmodified,* 147.

20. Caroline Whitbeck, "A Unitary Morality of Responsibility," unpublished paper, 22, ed. Eva Kittay and Diana Meyers.

21. H. Patricia Hynes, "Reconstructing Babylon: Women and Appropriate Technology" (Keynote address, Nordic Conference on Women, Environment, and Development, Norwegian Research Council for Science and the Humanities, the Secretariat for Women and Research, University of Oslo, Center for Research on Women, Oslo, Norway, November 1990), 59–60.

22. UNESCO Report on Social and Cultural Causes of Prostitution . . .". Division of Human Rights and Peace, 7.
23. Katha Pollitt, "The Strange Case of Baby M," *The Nation,* May 23, 1987, 688.
24. H. Patricia Hynes, *The Recurring Silent Spring* (New York: Pergamon Press, 1989), 162.
25. Hynes, *Recurring Silent Spring,* 163.